Programmed Therapy FOR STUTTERING in Children and Adults

Programmed Therapy FOR STUTTERING in Children and Adults

Third Printing

By

BRUCE P. RYAN, Ph.D.

Speech Pathologist
Research Associate
Behavioral Sciences Institute
Monterey, California
Formerly, Associate Professor
Speech Department
University of Oregon
Eugene, Oregon

THOMAS BOOKS · SYMBOL OF LEADERSHIP

CHARLES C THOMAS · PUBLISHER
Springfield · Illinois · U.S.A.

Published and Distributed Throughout the World by
CHARLES C THOMAS • PUBLISHER
Bannerstone House
301-327 East Lawrence Avenue, Springfield, Illinois, U.S.A.

ISBN 0-398-03100-2 (Cloth)
ISBN 0-398-03104-5 (Paper)

Library of Congress Catalog Card Number 73-20463

First Printing, 1974
Second Printing, 1977
Third Printing, 1980

With THOMAS BOOKS careful attention is given to all details of manufacturing and design. It is the Publisher's desire to present books that are satisfactory as to their physical qualities and artistic possibilities and appropriate for their particular use. THOMAS BOOKS will be true to those laws of quality that assure a good name and good will.

Printed in the United States of America
C-1

Library of Congress Cataloging in Publication Data
Ryan, Bruce P.
Programmed therapy for stuttering in children and adults.
Bibliography: p.
1. Speech disorders in children. 2. Speech therapy—Programmed instruction. 3. Speech, Disorders of. I. Title. [DNLM: 1. Stuttering—Therapy. WM475 R988p 1974]
RJ496.S7R9 616.8'554 73-20463
ISBN 0-398-03100-2

PREFACE

THIS IS A BOOK by a clinician interested in treating the problem of stuttering. The focus of this book is on therapy for people who stutter. Stuttering is viewed as learned behavior. The approach to therapy can be best characterized as behavior modification or contingency management or operant conditioning or programmed instruction. All of these systems draw from the same basic source of learning principles (Skinner, 1953; Honig, 1966; Bandura, 1969; Holland and Skinner, 1961).

There is much confusion today concerning the problem of stuttering and the "new technology" of behavior modification (Fraser, 1971). One purpose of this book is to present the *data* we have collected for evaluation and comparison. The book is essentially to share the past nine years of the author's experience in treating the problem of stuttering with fifty-eight people using a systematic behavioral technology. The data were collected at the University of Oregon and the Behavioral Sciences Institute. It is my hope that this sharing will permit all people interested in the problem of stuttering to appropriately evaluate this system and to help us all to cooperatively solve the problem of stuttering. This book may serve as a companion to the program book, *Programmed Conditioning for Fluency* (Ryan and Van Kirk, 1971).

The new behavioral technology suggests that one should limit himself to behaviors which he can systematically observe, count and manipulate. In the case of stuttering one of the behaviors of interest is the speech act. The major goal in this system is normal fluent speech. I realize that focussing only on the speech act appears to ignore the other dimensions of stuttering such as self-concept, avoidance, fear, psycho-social problems, etc. However, I am interested in many of these other aspects of stuttering and have commonly observed an improvement in them when the person has achieved normal fluent speech.

One may view the installation of fluent speech as only one of the many goals for people who stutter or he may look upon it as the single goal. I find no disagreement among experts that fluent speech for stutterers should be at least one of the goals of therapy. Stutterers themselves have unanimously requested fluent speech, although they have not all demonstrated this desire.

I purposely avoided a long introductory chapter on the principles of behavior modification because I felt that this information is well presented in many other sources (see bibliography). I did not provide an extensive review of either operant conditioning or stuttering itself for the same reason. Both Van Riper (1971) and Sheehan (1970) recently have provided extremely comprehensive, excellent reviews of the literature.

Rather, I chose to focus on the description of the procedures I have used and the results achieved with them. I have tried to make mostly data-bound statements, although I have also engaged in some speculation. I assume it will be clear to the reader when I am doing one or the other. You will find both failures and successes in this book and I hope you will learn from them as both my students and I did. We have been working cooperatively for the past nine years to achieve the best, most efficient, effective means of helping people who stutter.

The book is arranged with a very brief introductory Chapter I on stuttering and basic principles of operant analysis. Chapter II covers the mechanics of charting, counting, and computing stuttering rate. Chapter III describes evaluation. Chapter IV is on programming. Chapter V describes the four Establishment of Fluency Programs. Chapter VI discusses the Transfer and Maintenance Programs. Chapter VII contains discussion of individual client performance. Chapter VIII is a summary. The reader should not be surprised at finding some old techniques in new usages. Previous therapies have produced significant and lasting changes in some people who stutter. Systematic analysis simply permits one to select and organize procedures in a way which is helpful to the clinician and the client. It maximizes the probability that they will be successful.

My thanks to all those who have helped make this book possible: my colleagues; Dr. Charles Van Riper, Dr. George Shames, Dr. Donald Mowrer, Dr. Burl Gray; my students at the University of Oregon; Cheryl Lockard, Helen Fisher, Marilyn Howe, Denis Newman, Virginia Bingham, Linda Bragg, Bob Clay, Vincent Keane, Bob McCabe, Mary Lu Wilson, Suzanne Gowdy, Kathleen Griffin, Barbara Van Kirk, Barbara Mervo, Susan Trafton, Leslie Fisher, Bill De Mastus, Gerry Mill, Trudy Lewis, Brooke Belcher, Dia Graves, Kelly Timm, Carol Roland, Harriet Ellington, Jim Smith, Dave Miller, Dave Haugen, Margaret Wood, Marion Lea, Bonnie Moon, David Stenslen, Bill Worthley, Mary Ann Beggs, Meryl Synyshyn, Linda Backman, Marcia Harris, Virginia Brady, Emery Hildebrandt, Doris Butherus, Mary Grammacioni, Lloyd Guderjohn, Rita Bacon, Joanne Cooper, Eli Planedin, Lynn Kuhner, Judy Johanson, Don Robinson, Nancy Mullman, Marcia Smith, Craig Hull, and Reinhart Heurer, and finally, the people who stuttered with whom we worked. They taught us much about the problem and it is to them that this book is dedicated.

A final special thank you is due my family; Ardith, Jeff, Jim and Julie. They went about their lives while I spent nights and weekends writing this book. Without their love and understanding I would not have been able to do it.

B.P.R.

CONTENTS

Programmed Therapy
FOR STUTTERING
in Children and Adults

CHAPTER I

BEHAVIOR PRINCIPLES AND STUTTERING

BEHAVIOR: OPERANT AND RESPONDENT

OPERANT ANALYSIS IS A FORM of behaviorism, a system for analyzing and controlling our environment. A number of terms have been used to identify this system such as behavior modification, precision teaching, programmed instruction, operant conditioning, functional analysis of behavior and the experimental analysis of behavior, among others. All of these procedures have similar basic principles most of which are derived from the work of Skinner (1938; 1953; 1957) and described extensively in many other books such as those by Bandura (1969), Krasner and Ullmann (1965) and Honig (1966). The approach is characterized by the methodology of (1) direct observation, (2) continuous measurement and (3) systematic manipulation of behavior. It has been applied to many behaviors (Bradfield, 1971; Brookshire, 1967; Fargo, Behrns, and Nolen, 1970; Giradeau and Spradlin, 1970; Holland, 1967; and Sloane and MacAuley, 1968).

In this system all behavior may be divided into two classes: (1) respondent behavior—that behavior which is under the control of specific stimuli, is generally covert (e.g. glandular activity, simple reflexes, anxiety, autonomic nervous system functioning) and (2) operant behavior—that behavior which is brought under the control of varying stimuli by the consequences which follow its occurrence and which is generally overt (e.g. striped muscle activity, central nervous system functioning, speech, stuttering). Operant behavior is controlled by its consequences.

It is this system of analysis of human behavior which was used to develop programs of therapy for people who stutter.

STUTTERING

There are many definitions of stuttering. Most of them include reference to broken or stuttered speech, special fears or anxiety about talking and self-concept or attitudes relating to both fear of talking and/or disordered talking itself. The causes for stuttering may be grouped into three categories: physiological (due to a number of different physiological problems), learned (any number of behaviors and/or attitudes may be learned) and psychodynamic (the root of all stuttering is personal maladjustment). Although the research is not yet definitive at this point there appears to be much interest and value in viewing stuttering as learned behavior (Sheehan, 1970; Shames, 1970; Van Riper, 1971; Gregory, 1968; Goldiamond, 1965).

Stuttering as learned behavior is composed of both operant and respondent responses. A number of studies have clearly demonstrated that much of stuttering is operant behavior (Flanagan, Goldiamond and Azrin, 1958; Goldiamond, 1965; Martin and Siegel, 1966a; 1966b; and Ryan, 1964). Brutten and Shoemaker (1967) have discussed in great detail the possible respondent components of stuttering. There remains some question both as to the relative importance of the operant and respondent aspects of stuttering and to the extent of their interrelationships (Shames, 1969a; 1970; Van Riper, 1971; Goldiamond, 1965; Sheehan, 1970; Skinner, 1957; Gray and England, 1972; Gray, 1969; Shames and Sherrick, 1963; 1965). This does not preclude the possibility that stuttering may have a physiological basis nor that many people who stutter are emotionally disturbed. Neither of these possibilities, however, may have much relevance to the development of fluency training programs.

Stuttering is composed of three classes of behavior: a speech act, an anxiety component, and an attitude which is expressed by verbal statements by the person about himself or herself and his or her speech problem. The speech part of stuttering behavior refers to the activities of the oral and breathing mechanisms. Words and parts of words are repeated, prolonged and said with tension. The breath is held. There are often long pauses. Words are said with extreme tension and struggle. It is possible for this behavior to occur in any speaker at any time. This is the common, visible component of stuttering. It is of interest to note that this behavior can occur in isolation, i.e. without either undue anxiety or verbal statements concerning the existence of *stuttering* or the self-concept of one as a *stutterer.*

The anxiety part of stuttering refers to the activities of the autonomic nervous system. Excitement is similar to, if not the same as anxiety. Anxiety is not overt. It can be sensed or measured only indirectly through certain physiological correlates such as palmar sweat or through interviewing the person. Anxiety or excitement about speaking may exist in isolation, i.e. without either deviation in speech or a concept of stuttering.

In an effort to find the cause of stuttering, to describe it fully and to eventually develop a therapy to treat it there have been many speculations, and some research, about the various interrelationships among these three behavioral classes of stuttering. Mathematically, there are numerous possible cause-effect interrelationships, but for the purposes of this discussion I have limited them to only three. These are shown in Figure 1.

Anxiety Produces Stuttering

There has been much written in the literature and much research about anxiety and stuttering (Van Riper, 1971; Sheehan, 1970). Most of it suggests that anxiety produces stuttering. Stuttering is developed because the person was made anxious or stuttering was evoked in the presence of anxiety. If this is true, treatment of stuttering lies in elimination of the anxiety. There is a paucity of data to support this notion, although much discussion has been made of it (Gray, 1969; Goldiamond, 1965; Gray and England, 1972).

Attitudes Produce Anxiety and Stuttering

This is a procedure whereby people with self-concept problems or emotional disturbance generate anxiety which in turn generates stuttering. If the person has a poor self-value system or an emotional disturbance he would be likely to stutter. If this is true, therapy would focus on improving attitude or emotional adjustment. Psychotherapy or any form of talk therapy would

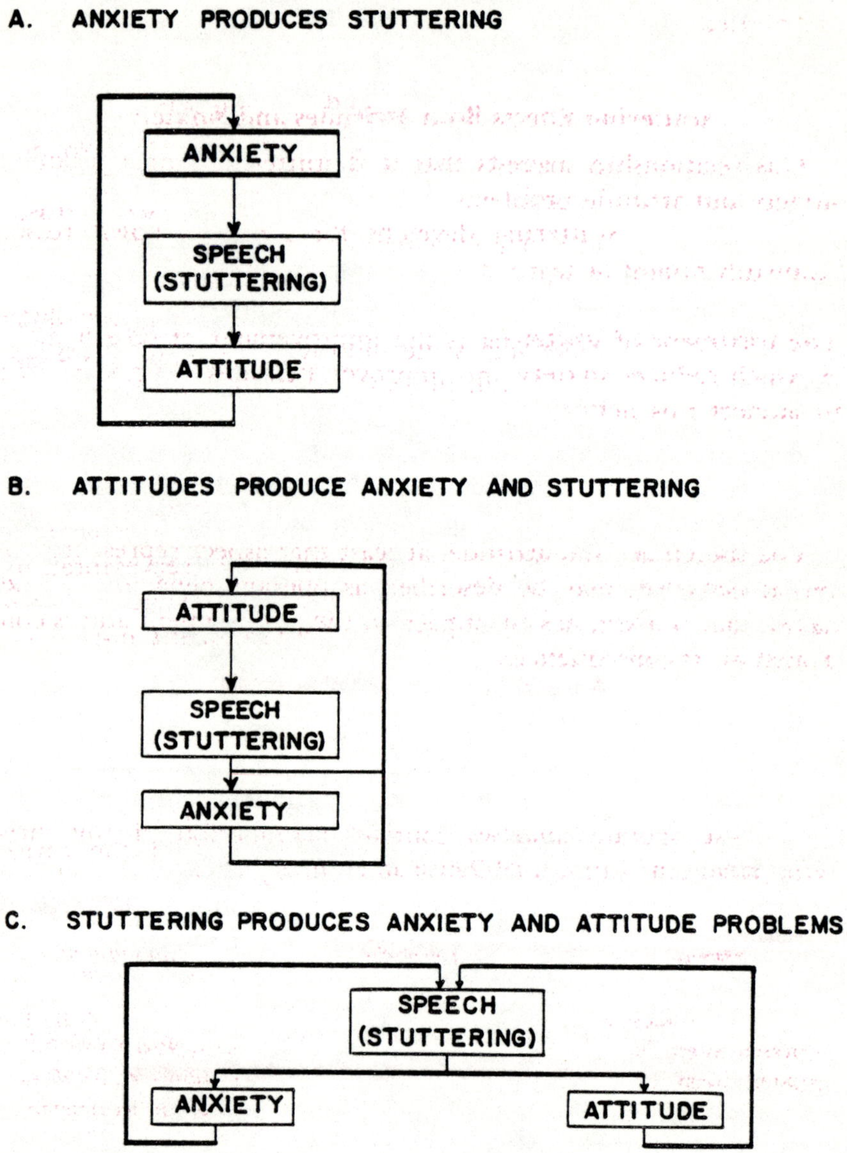

Figure 1. Three inter-relationships among speech, anxiety and attitude factors in stuttering behavior.

be the treatment process. There is a paucity of data to support this notion, although much discussion has been made of it (Sheehan, 1970).

Stuttering Effects Both Attitudes and Anxiety

This relationship suggests that it is stuttering which produces anxiety and attitude problems. A person's behavior influences the concept of self. Stuttering develops for some unknown reason (probably taught or learned, Shames and Sherrick, 1963) and two of the aftermath experiences are anxiety and attitude problems. The treatment of stuttering is the improvement of speech fluency which reduces anxiety and improves attitudes. There are data to support this notion (Goldiamond, 1965; Shames, 1970; Ryan, 1971; Martin and Haroldson, 1969).

OPERANT ASPECTS OF STUTTERING

The speech act and attitude, at least that aspect represented by verbal behavior, may be described as operant behavior, i.e. behavior that is overt, has an impact on the environment and is controlled by its consequences.

Speech

Of the two operant aspects of stuttering, speech and attitude, let us first examine speech and its analysis within the operant system. Most operant analyses contain examination of the three term paradigm; stimuli, response and consequence (sometimes referred to as reinforcer, punisher, S+, R_f, R+, etc.).

Stimuli	*Response*	*Consequence*
Any verbal or nonverbal event which evokes or is present when the response is emitted	Any verbal or nonverbal behavior which occurs in the presence of or after the stimuli have been presented	Any verbal or nonverbal event which occurs after the response and has influence on its probability of occurrence

An illustration of operant stuttering analysis would be:

Stimuli	*Response*	*Consequence*
A book	Read aloud and stutter	"Thank you for reading."

Other possible stimuli are:

Stimuli	*Response*	*Consequence*
Instructions to read A book A clinician	Read aloud and stutter	"Thank you," etc.

A deeper analysis of the response class would yield:

Stimuli	*Response*	*Consequences*
Instructions, etc.	100 words read 27 stuttered words 3 minutes to read	"Thank you," etc.

Additional different consequences could be:

Stimuli	*Response*	*Consequences*
Instructions, etc.	Read aloud	Nodding ("yes") Looking away Yawning "Thank you," etc.

Thus far we have been analyzing a fairly common situation in stuttering therapy. The stutterer is asked to read, does so and the clinician reacts (provides consequences). The consequence may increase the behavior, decrease it or have no effect at all. We can decide the valance or power of the consequence by observing its effect. Table I shows an analysis of consequent events.

Using this table, we can determine the probable effects of various events; knowing the effects, we can name the process; and knowing the process, we can predict the effect.

The common measure of response strength is frequency. Each

TABLE I

CONSEQUENT EVENTS, PROCESSES AND EFFECTS IN OPERANT ANALYSIS

Event	*Administer*		*Withdraw*	
	Name of process	Effect	Name of process	Effect
Positive event	Positive reinforcement (acceleration)	Increase	Punishment II Extinction (deceleration)	Decrease
Aversive or negative event	Punishment I (deceleration)	Decrease	Negative reinforcement (acceleration)	Increase

occurrence of a behavior under direct observation is counted. Frequency is usually measured over time which yields a rate, e.g. ten responses per minute. Changes, increase or decrease, in rate indicate that evoking stimuli and/or consequences have been changed and have affected response rate.

Now that we have analyzed an ongoing situation, we can next examine altering the evoking stimuli and/or the consequences to bring about a change in behavior (this may be called therapy). A change in stimuli or instructions would be:

Stimuli	*Response*	*Consequence*	*(Effect)*
Instructions, etc. plus, "Read very slowly and as fluently as you can."	Read	"Very good"	Stuttering decreases

We may infer that our instructions were stimuli which evoked less stuttering and more fluency. We can control stuttering operants by manipulating the evoking stimuli.

A manipulation of the consequence would be:

Stimuli	*Response*	*Consequence*	*(Effect)*
Instructions, etc.	Reading aloud	"No, don't do that" (after each stuttered word)	Stuttering decreases

From this example we may infer that our consequence of, "No," was a punishing event because the stuttering decreased. We can control stuttering by manipulating consequences.

A final factor in the analysis of consequences is the schedule on which they are provided. Different schedules produce different results as is shown in Table II.

TABLE II

THE ESTABLISHMENT AND MAINTENANCE EFFECTS OF THREE DIFFERENT SCHEDULES OF REINFORCEMENT

Schedule	*Effect Establishment of a Response*	*Effect Maintenance of a Response*
100% fixed ratio or interval	Excellent	Poor
50% fixed or variable ratio or interval	Fair	Fair
10% fixed or variable ratio or interval	Poor	Excellent

As can be seen in Table II, a 100 per cent continuous schedule is optimal when a response is first being taught or acquired. After it has been learned fairly well the schedule should be changed to a leaner one such as 50 per cent. Finally, when the response is quite well learned the reinforcement schedule contains very few reinforcers. Most normal human social behavior in the world is maintained by very lean schedules of social reinforcement.

Next, let us examine some of the different consequences and their possible effects on stuttering behavior.

Stimuli	*Response*	*Consequences*	*(Effects)*
Instructions, etc.	Read aloud	Nodding (yes)	Stuttering increases
Instructions, etc.	Read aloud	Looking away	Stuttering decreases
Instructions, etc.	Read aloud	Yawning	No effect

Hence, we may infer (see Table I) that *nodding* is positively reinforcing because it increases the responses, *looking away* is punishing because it decreases the responses, and *yawning* is neutral because it has no effect. Shames and Sherrick (1963) suggest that stuttering is maintained on complex schedules of both negative and positive reinforcement.

Attitudes

The second operant aspect of stuttering, attitude (as defined by verbal statements) is not so easily handled. One behavioristic approach to this problem is exemplified by Shames (1969b; 1970) and Rhodes, Shames and Egolf (1971) who have manipulated the types of verbal statements the stutterer makes with the result being increased fluency. Another interesting aspect is the finding by Shames (1969b) and Martin and Haroldson (1969) that the attainment of fluent speech produced positive verbal statements and attitude changes. Using a combined approach Blind, Shames and Egolf (1971) were able to manipulate both attitudes and speech.

RESPONDENT ASPECTS OF STUTTERING

Let us turn now to an analysis of respondent components of stuttering. The essential one is anxiety. Respondents and operants not only occur simultaneously, but they may evoke or elicit or even interfere with each other (Skinner, 1953; 1957) or they may be completely independent of each other (Gray and England, 1972). Most studies of the experimental analysis of stuttering behavior do not include respondent behavior such as anxiety mainly because it is so difficult to observe, hence measure, hence manipulate (Goldiamond, 1965). An analysis of the respondent aspects of stuttering would contain only two terms: stimulus and response.

Stimulus	*Response*
Any conditioned or unconditioned stimulus which elicits a response	Any response which is consistently elicited by a stimulus

An illustration of this would be:

Stimulus	*Response*
A large audience (assume a request to speak to the audience)	Anxiety (increased heart rate and palmer sweating)

Most of the literature of stuttering as exemplified in the writings of Van Riper (1971), Sheehan (1970) and Brutten and Shoemaker (1967), describes in great detail the assumed anxiety components of stuttering. Therefore, there is no need to repeat that information here.

THE FOCUS OF THIS BOOK

In viewing behavior we can analyze it in terms of stimuli, responses and consequences. We can observe ongoing behavior to determine what is occurring or we can manipulate variables to bring about changes in behavior. The effect of a stimulus or a consequence is determined by observing and measuring the response and then manipulating either or both the stimuli and consequences. Schedules of consequences (reinforcement) are important in establishing, and maintaining behavior. Behaviorists develop operational definitions or descriptions of the behavior so that they may pinpoint it and measure it reliably. Stuttered and fluent speech are overt and can be measured. Operational definitions to aid in discrimination between stuttered and fluent speech can be made. Anxiety and attitudes are not so easily measured.

Although it may be argued that any really effective approach to stuttering must include modification of speech, anxiety and attitude (Blind, Shames and Egolf, 1971), the data coming out of the operant/clinic-laboratory seem to indicate that the production of fluent speech alone tends to bring about concurrent changes in anxiety and attitude. In other words, to modify the attitudes and anxiety of the person who stutters, the best procedure is to provide him or her with the capability of speaking fluently. An operant analysis appears to permit and encourage the achievement of this goal. The focus of this book is on stuttering and fluency as operant speech acts subject to control by the consequences they generate.

SUMMARY

This short introductory chapter described both operant and respondent aspects of stuttering with an emphasis on the operant. Stuttering is viewed as a problem concerning the three behavioral classes of stuttered speech, anxiety and attitude. The emphasis in this book is on stuttered and fluent speech as the operant behaviors of interest.

CHAPTER II

THE MECHANICS OF OPERANT PROCEDURES

THE MECHANICS OF OPERANT PROCEDURES to work with the problem of stuttering concern response definition, counting stuttered and fluent words, reliability of judgments, timing, computing the rate of stuttering, the rate of talking, charting and scoring.

THE TARGET BEHAVIOR

As stated in Chapter I the focus in this book is on the motor speech acts of fluency and stuttering. It becomes important to define the basic unit of target behavior. Historically, in the operant experimentation it has been the stuttered word (Goldiamond, 1960a; 1960b; 1962; 1965; Ryan, 1969; Shames, 1969a). This has proved adequate although some authorities prefer the stuttered syllable which permits more finite counting of stuttering within multisyllabic words (Ingham and Andrews, 1971). Still others have used the stuttering moment or time units of fluency. The work reported in this book and the system to be discussed have employed the stuttered word and the fluent word as the basic behavioral units.

DEFINITION OF THE STUTTERED WORD

In developing the present set of working definitions of stuttered words we started with the classical Johnson (1961) categories of disfluencies and modified his original eight categories to yield the nine found in Table III.

It is necessary to differentiate between normal disfluencies and stuttered words. Analysis of the speech of both normal speakers and people referred to as stutterers has consistently shown over-

TABLE III

TYPES OF DISFLUENCIES AND STUTTERED WORDS AND EXAMPLES

Types	*Examples*	*Exceptions*
A. Normal disfluencies		
1. Interjections	"uh, well, um, mmm"	If it occurs at a high rate. Consistent occurrence as a starter for a stuttered word.
2. Revisions	"I rent-went . . ."	If it occurs at a high rate. If the first sounds of a commonly stuttered word are said and then revised.
3. Incomplete phrases	"I went-she found . . ."	If it occurs at a high rate. If parts of a stuttered word are said and then the next different phrase is said.
4. Phrase repetition	"I went, I went . . ."	Could be a starter device. If it occurs at high rate. If stuttered word follows it.
5. Pause	"I (pause) went . . ."	If it occurs at a high rate. If it is accompanied by unusual facial movements or grimaces or fixed mouth postures. If unusually long or in unusual places.
B. Stuttered words		
6. Whole-word repetitions	"I, I went . . ."	If it occurs at low rate and is composed of only single repetitions. If each word is separated by a pause.
7. Part-word repetitions	"I w-w-w-went . . . I w-I went . . ."	
8. Prolongations	"I weeeeeeeeent . . ."	
9. Struggle	Any of the preceding stuttered words or normal disfluencies accompanied by struggle. Any secondary characteristic such as tongue protrusion, facial grimaces immediately preceding the utterance of a word.	

lap (Johnson, 1961) i.e. both stuttered words and normal disfluencies occur in the speech of both normally fluent speakers and people who stutter. It is the relative frequency of occurrence of these behaviors (or at least of certain types of them) which differentiates the stutterer from the nonstutterer.

In Table III the list of nine types of disfluencies includes five patterns (1-5) which are commonly thought of as normal disfluencies and four patterns (6-9) which are commonly classified as stuttering behavior. Pattern 6 (whole word repetitions) is difficult to classify because there are several sub-forms such as "went to . . . to the" with a pause in between the two "to's". There is also variation in the frequency of repetitions from one repetition, "my-my" to several, "my-my-my-my. . . ." After observing many people who stuttered we have decided to routinely count whole word repetitions as stuttered words. We believe it was better to err in the direction of over defining rather than under defining. With some people who stutter it may be helpful to use a category called "other," in which one describes some stuttering behavior which does not fit neatly into one of the categories. For example, audible inhalations or tongue protrusions, may be described as "other" stuttering behaviors. Commonly, we have put them in the category of struggle.

There are many different systems one might use to classify moments of stuttering or types of stuttered words. Brutten and Shoemaker (1970) suggest that ninety-seven different classifications of behavior are necessary to cover the verbal and nonverbal components of stuttering. Wingate's standard definition (1964) was modified into twelve classes by Hood (1971). Shames et al. (1970) developed a classification system composed of fourteen behaviors. The reduction of these extensive classes to only four types of stuttered words: whole word repetitions, part-word repetitions, prolongations and struggle, has proved to be adequate to permit analysis and elimination of stuttering behavior in the people with whom we have worked.

It is possible to group all forms of disfluencies and stutterings under three categories: additions (1,2,3,5,9); repetitions (4,6,7) and prolongations (8). This grouping may be helpful to the clinician beginning to learn to recognize various types of stuttered words.

IDENTIFYING AND COUNTING STUTTERED WORDS

The stuttered word is defined as the occurrence of one or more stuttering behaviors immediately preceding or occurring concurrently with the production of a given word. The basic decision is binary. A given word is perceived as either stuttered or not. Each stuttered word is counted only once. The time space described is that from the final phoneme of the preceding word to the final phoneme of the word under scrutiny. Hence, it is possible that many different behaviors may occur before the word being examined is finally spoken. It is still counted as only one stuttered word.

Examples of *one* stuttered word:

(a) c-c-c-ar
(b) c-car, c-ar
(c) (tongue protrusion, exhalation of air) c-c-c-c-c-aaaaaaaar

The definition of stuttered words (deciding what we will count) begins with obtaining a sample of the speech behavior of the person who stutters. The clinician must then decide which behaviors to count, usually whole word repetitions, part-word repetitions, prolongations and struggle behaviors. Arriving at this decision may require viewing or listening to the collected sample several times. Tape recordings, especially video tape recordings, are helpful. Once we decide on our definitions, we must be consistent about what we count.

Try your skill at counting stuttered words in this utterance: (The answers follow.)

A. "Th-th-this is not ah, not ah very hard sssssssample to count, but y-but you should still be careful about your, about the way you classify each, each of the (pause) disfluencies, because, because some of them are (struggle) normal and don't count as stuttered words." Number of SW . . . . . .

Check your score and then try this one.

B. "Some pe-people have very set-subtle stuttering bb-behaviors such as ccccccircumlocution and sub-sub-substitution. These aaare extremely difficult, extremely difficult to detect, de-de-define and to (struggle) objectively count. Look, look for oooooovert signs." Number of SW . . . . . .

Check your score and then try this one.

C. "The hardest p-part of counting is w-when the person has improved his stuttering (exhalation) so much that, that, that there are only ssssmall traces of his f-former problem. Uh, uh, most of his present disfluencies are nar, normal, b-but he has the, has the reputation of being a stutterer and th-th-th-th-th-that is h-h-ard to lllive down." Number of SW . . . . . .

Answers to above:

A. Stuttered words = 7—"this, sample, you, very, each, because, normal."

B. Stuttered words = 9—"People, behaviors, circumlocution, substitution, are, define, objectively, look, overt."

C. Stuttered words = 10—"part, when, so, that, small, former, but, that, hard, live."

Shames (1971) suggested that if one could get a stenographer to carefully transcribe the speech of a person who stutters, the task of counting stuttered words would be greatly reduced. Unfortunately, the task of clinical management of stuttering requires immediate decisions about whether or not any given word was stuttered. Clinicians often use mechanical counters or simply make a pencil mark for each stuttered word observed. For further practice, the reader may wish to listen to a tape recording which will aid in learning how to count stuttered words (Ryan and Van Kirk, 1973).

The advantages of this binary counting system are that there is a high reliability in counting and it is quite easy to teach beginners, including the client, to count. The major disadvantage is that this is a gross count and may not accurately reflect important changes in the client's stuttering. For example, a client who demonstrated a great number of struggle stuttered words may change (improve) to whole word repetitions and the count would remain the same. There is an improvement or change, but simple counting does not show it. The number of stuttered words may be constant while the type of stuttering changes. In a few of our cases, the frequency of stuttering actually increased as the client developed a different, simpler, more efficient stuttering pattern. Later we will discuss the counting of total words to help solve this problem.

TOPOGRAPHICAL ANALYSIS

A topographical analysis of a stuttering behavior is a classification of the different types of stuttering behavior. This helps the clinician make a decision about severity. For example, a child with a high frequency of struggle behaviors would be evaluated as more severe than a child with an equally high frequency of whole word repetitions. Careful topographical analyses of stuttering can be helpful to the clinician to decide whom to take for training, to determine progress and to decide when to dismiss a client.

The topography of stuttering may also have certain prognostic value. This has not been studied carefully enough yet to know much about it. Do certain forms of stuttering condition or decondition more than others? For example, do part-word repetitions like "c-c-c-ar," respond differently to conditioning from part-word repetitions like "that c, that car." Brutten and Shoemaker (1967) suggest different forms of stuttering may have different histories of reinforcement, and that they may also be either operant or respondent responses or "fluency failures."

Another aspect of topographical analysis concerns secondary characteristics. They are usually overlaid on the speech behavior. By eliminating the *oral* part of stuttering we have observed that the secondaries, such as arm swinging, eye blinking, head rolling, tongue protrusion, etc., have disappeared without special attention drawn to them. We generally count secondary behaviors as struggle behaviors occurring concurrently with stuttered words.

RELIABILTY OF JUDGMENTS

The consistency or reliability of judgments concerning stuttered words is important. One form of checking is to compare counts with an observer. Another way is for one observer to count on two different occasions. The sample to be counted should be tape recorded. To aid in this process, the Stuttering Description and Reliability Form shown in Figure 2 may be used.

THE UPPER PART, SECTION A. Description of Topography of Stuttering, contains the common four categories of whole word repetition, part-word repetition, prolongation and struggle. There is a space to check the presence of a particular type. There are also extra blanks to name additional types such as the other disfluencies (phase repetition at a high rate, for example) or to enumerate special forms of struggle behavior such as tongue protrusion, head turning, and exhalation of air. In the second column, the frequency of each of the forms is counted for one-minute samples. A sample of one minute in length has been adequate for this purpose. There is a place for reading, monologue, and conversation.

THE LOWER PART, SECTION B. Reliability, is to aid in achieving agreement with another person and to calibrate the ability to count stuttered words correctly. Independent counts are desirable. The observers listen separately to the tape recording or shield their counting activities from each other. To check a single observer's count, the observer may listen to the tape one day, wait a day or so and do it again without looking at the results of the first count. This is continued during one-minute segments until 90 per cent agreement or higher on two consecutive segments has been achieved. If there is difficulty in reaching 90 per cent agreement, it is necessary to redefine more clearly or discuss with the observer what is being counted.

The purpose of the reliability check is to insure accurate counting of the appropriate behaviors. This procedure helps to insure correct decisions about which words are stuttered. It may be extremely helpful when working with clients whose stuttering is very subtle or extremely rapid.

Another variation is to repeat this same process with the client (usually older children or adults). Stuttered word identification is the first step in several training programs. The process described above may be used to achieve the goal of correct stuttering identification by the client. The client becomes Observer No. 2.

STUTTERING DESCRIPTION AND RELIABILITY FORM

Client: ________ Clinician (1) ________

Date: ________ Observer/Listener (2) ________

A. Description of Topography of Stuttering

Types—(Each stuttered word classified only once)	If Present Check	Read. Rate per ___ Min. Sample	Total	Monologue Rate Per ___ Min. Sample	Total
Whole Word Repetition					
Part Word Repetition					
Prolongation					
Struggle					
Other: (Describe and Name Other Forms)					

Figure 2a

To determine the percentage of agreement, a ratio is derived from the number of stuttered words counted by the clinician compared to the number of stuttered words counted by another observer. The smaller number is always put in the numerator position.

Example:

$$\frac{\text{Clinician's count} \quad 10}{\text{Other person's count} \quad 12} \times 100 = 83\%$$

B. Reliability ____Live ____Audio Tape ____Video Tape

Number of Minutes and Percentage of Agreement

Mode	1 Minute (1) obs 1	obs 2	%	1 Minute (2) obs 1	obs 2	%	1 Minute (3) obs 1	obs 2	%	1 Minute (4) obs 1	obs 2	%
Reading												
Monologue												
Conversation												

Figure 2b

Figure 2. Stuttering Description and Reliability Form.

Try these: (The answers will follow.)

A. Clinician's count / Other person's count $\frac{48}{57} \times 100 =$ . . %

B. Other person's count / Clinician's count $\frac{23}{30} \times 100 =$ . . %

Answer A: 84%.

Answer B: 77%.

TIMING

It is necessary to time the talking and reading of the client as part of the mechanics of conducting programmed therapy. A stopwatch is mandatory. The basic rule is to time all the talking of the client, including the blocks. If there are short pauses, it will be difficult to stop and start the stopwatch fast enough, so let it continue. If longer pauses occur, then do stop the watch. A stopwatch which has a control for stopping and then continuing on from where it was stopped is preferable to one that resets to the beginning after each time it is stopped. We have found that running a stopwatch during the training becomes very automatic after some practice with it. The clinician soon learns to carry on quite a normal conversation while automatically starting and stopping the stopwatch to time only the speech of the client. The clinician is also counting stuttered words while timing. The time of talking and the number of stuttered words are then used to compute the rate of stuttering.

THE RATE OF STUTTERING

Thus far we have talked about defining stuttered words, counting them, and timing the talking act. Our count represents the frequency of occurrence. We now want to add the time dimension to yield a rate of stuttering or stuttered words per minute (SW/M).

$$\text{SW/M (Stuttered Words Per Minute)} = \frac{\text{Number of Stuttered Words}}{\text{Time (Minutes)}}$$

Example:

$$\frac{\text{15 Stuttered Words}}{\text{10 Minutes}} = 1.5 \text{ SW/M}$$

Try these: (The answers will follow.)

A. $$\frac{\text{25 SW}}{\text{3 Minutes}} = \ldots\text{SW/M}$$

B. $$\frac{\text{15 SW}}{\text{18 Minutes}} = \ldots\text{SW/M}$$

Answer A. 8.3̲3̲ SW/M.

Answer B. .8̲3̲ SW/M.

The computation of rate permits us to compare samples with different time bases. Rate is the simplest measure of response strength or learning (Skinner, 1953). We count stuttered words and time the client's talking time throughout all of our work. We have a constant measure of stuttering rate which helps us evaluate progress and the effects of the procedures we are using. Simple rate computers are described by Branch and Sulzbacher (1968) and Fargo and Behrns (1969). The Percentage Finder developed by Thompson and Carlston (1961) may also be used to determine rate.

THE RATE OF TALKING

We also measure the rate of talking or words read or spoken over time. The rules are: 1) count each word produced so that in whole word repetitions, phrase repetitions and revisions we would count each word and 2) do not count interjections. An example of these rules in action:

"I went, went to the store to find a wheel for my, for my uh
1 2 3 4 5 6 7 8 9 10 11 12 13 14
b-b-brother who doesn't, didn't know where to find them."
15 16 17 18 19 20 21 22 23

There are twenty-three words in this sample when each word produced is counted according to the two rules. The total number of words read or spoken is then divided by the time to derive words read per minute (WR/M) or words spoken per minute (WS/M).

$$\begin{array}{l} \text{WR/M (Words Read per Minute)} \\ \qquad\qquad \text{or} \\ \text{WS/M (Words Spoken per Minute)} \end{array} = \frac{\text{Number of Words}}{\text{Time (Minutes)}}$$

Example:

$$\frac{\text{150 Words}}{\text{3 Minutes}} = \text{50 Words Read or Spoken per Minute (WR or WS/M)}$$

Try these: (The answers will follow.)

A. $$\frac{\text{200 Words Read}}{\text{2 Minutes}} = \ldots\ldots \text{WR/M}$$

B. $$\frac{\text{170 Words Spoken}}{\text{5 Minutes}} = \ldots\ldots \text{WS/M}$$

Answer A. 100.0 WS/M
Answer B. 34.0 WS/M

CHARTING

After rates have been figured it is important to store and display this information. The rates in stuttered words per minute (SW/M) are put on a chart (some people prefer the word, *graph*). The chart has the number of stuttered words along the ordinate and the number of sessions or days on the abscissa.

Example:

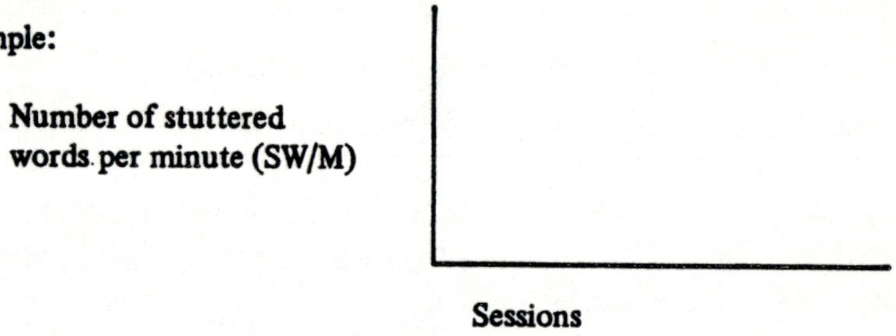

Diagram 1

Hence 10 SW/M in session one, 7 SW/M in session two and 13 SW/M in session three would look like this on the chart with "X's" representing each rate.

Example:

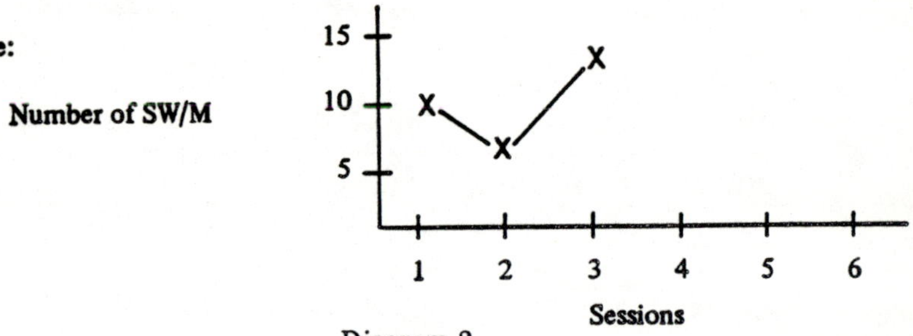

Diagram 2

Words read or spoken per minute (WR or WS/M) may also be charted in this manner.

The visual record of the varying rates is helpful to both the clinician and the client. Any regular charting or graphing paper may be used. However, there are some special ones like that by Lindsley (1968). He developed a 6-cycle logarithmic chart which permits the recording of rates of .0001 to 1000 responses per minute to be shown on the same paper. Of interest to those working with the problem of stuttering is the area under 1 SW/M. Most operant programs of therapy will produce reductions to 1 SW/M or less, but the stuttering behavior may continue to exist at some strength under 1 SW/M. The logarithmic chart paper permits examination of the under 1 SW/M rate. Another universal chart is offered by Johnston (1970).

Mowrer (1969; 1971a) described 2 and 3-cycle logarithmic charts. An example of a 4-cycle logarithmic chart which covers 0 through 300 responses per minute is shown in Figure 3. This range is adequate to permit the recording of speech behaviors including stuttering and talking rates. A coding of "X" for reading, "Δ" for monologue and "0" for conversation is used so that one would know which mode the client was working in for the rate displayed.

Additional information which is helpful to have on the chart is the name or number of the step of the program on which the client is working. With that information the clinician can recreate the clinical session.

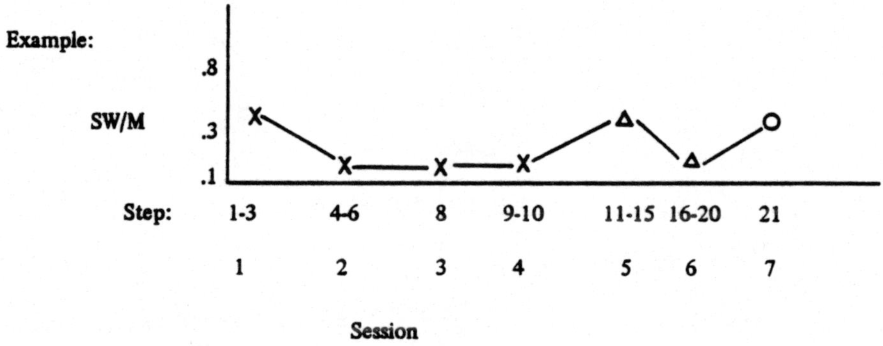

Diagram 3

We have used both forms of chart (linear and 2,4 and 6 cycle logarithmic). We like the logarithmic charts as they help us understand better what is happening below 1 SW/M. We like the Lindsley (1968) 6 cycle especially because it permits the recording of data for twenty weeks or half a school year on one page and it is extremely sensitive to the under one per minute rate data. It does not, however, have enough room to list all the pro-

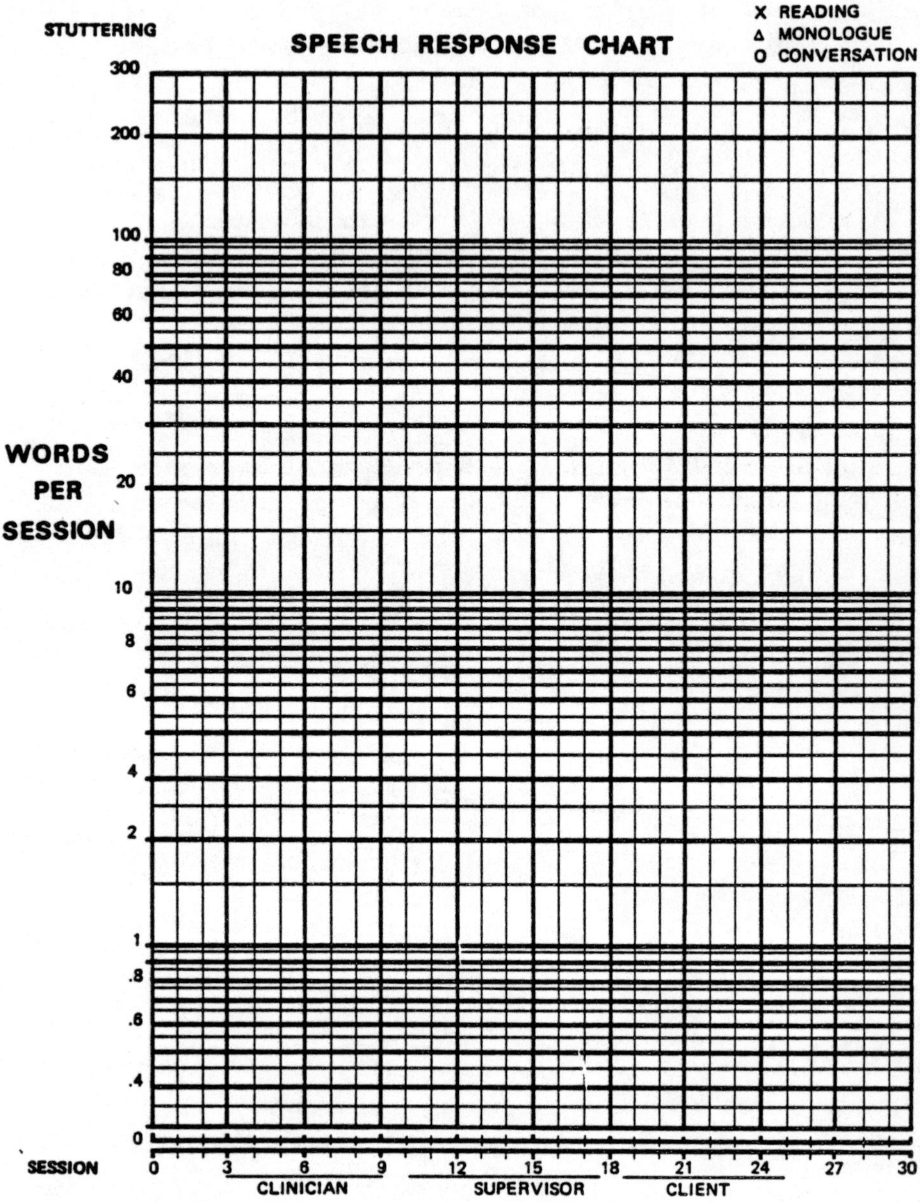

Figure 3. 4-Cycle Speech Response Chart (Reprinted with permission from Donald Mowrer, Arizona State University, Tempe, Arizona).

gram steps that the client went through each day. The Johnston (1970) chart appears to hold much promise.

Charts serve different purposes. For research and the development of programs the more complex charts such as Lindsley's and Johnston's are extremely valuable and we have used them. However, for clinical use we recommend one like the one shown in Figure 4.

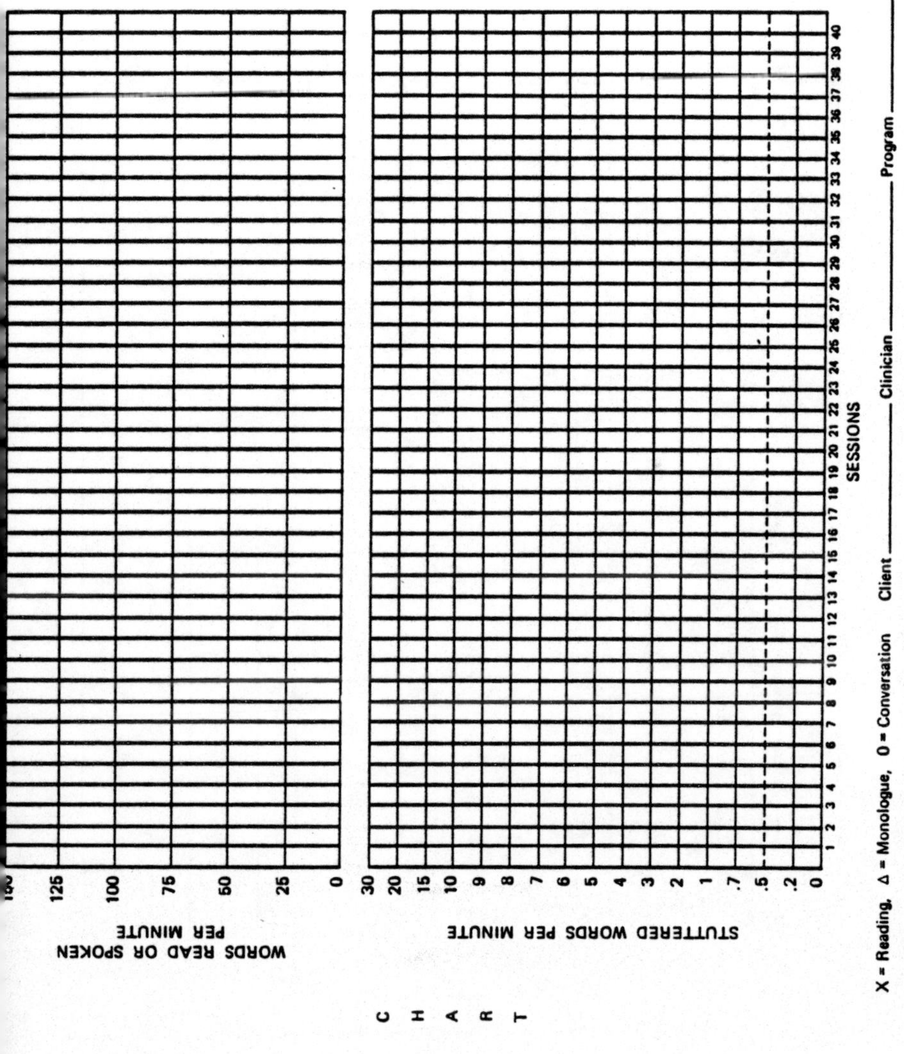

Figure 4. Chart (Reprinted with permission from Behavioral Sciences Institute, Monterey, California, copyright, 1971).

DATA SHEET Sheet Number:________ Name:________________

Date	Session	Step	Tape	Time (Minutes)	Words Read or Spoken–Total	WS/M WR/M	Words Stuttered Total			SW/M Per Step	Session Total SW/M	Comments
							Clinician	Client	%			

Figure 5. Data Sheet (Reprinted with permission from Behavioral Sciences Institute, Monterey, California, copyright, 1971).

This chart is designed to show a range of 0 to 30 SW/M. It gives special space to the rate under 1 SW/M. There is room to list the program step numbers. In the top portion can be listed word rate. The chart is simple enough for the client to easily view and understand the progress made.

RECORDING DATA

Another method of recording data is on a data sheet. We use this form with most programs. It is shown in Figure 5. The basic information about a session is shown on the data sheet. It aids the clinician in keeping track of where the client is in the program and current data. Data points such as SW/M are taken off this data sheet and transferred to the chart. We use this data sheet with all of our programs.

SCORING

A rather common procedure in the operant system is scoring. Scoring refers to recording the accuracy of responses emitted by the client. Not all therapy programs are scored in this manner, only Establishment Programs 1 and 4 and parts of the Transfer Program. A common scoring form is shown in Figure 6. There is basic identifying information at the top of the form. The numbered blanks are used to fill in either "X" or "/" for correct or "0" for wrong. The symbol "X" means the client was correct and received a special reinforcer while "/" means the client was correct but received no special reinforcer (this occurs commonly when on a 50 per cent or less schedule of reinforcement). The percentage of correct responses may be computed.

Example:

$$\frac{\text{Number Correct}}{\text{Total}} \quad \frac{(X + /)}{(X + / + 0)} \times 100 = \ldots\ldots\% \text{ Correct}$$

$$\frac{30}{40} \times 100 = 75\% \text{ Correct}$$

On it we can keep track of the correct responses ("X's"), the number of stuttered words ("0's") and the time, which we write above the line.

SCORE SHEET

PROGRAM ____________________

CRITERION ____________________

DATE ____________________

TIME __________ TO __________

1	2	3	4	5	6	7	8	9	10	11	12	13	14	15	16	17	18	19	20	TOTALS
																				X/ ______
21	22	23	24	25	26	27	28	29	30	31	32	33	34	35	36	37	38	39	40	X/O ______
																				% ______

1	2	3	4	5	6	7	8	9	10	11	12	13	14	15	16	17	18	19	20	
																				X/ ______
21	22	23	24	25	26	27	28	29	30	31	32	33	34	35	36	37	38	39	40	X/O ______
																				% ______

1	2	3	4	5	6	7	8	9	10	11	12	13	14	15	16	17	18	19	20	
																				X/ ______
21	22	23	24	25	26	27	28	29	30	31	32	33	34	35	36	37	38	39	40	X/O ______
																				% ______

1	2	3	4	5	6	7	8	9	10	11	12	13	14	15	16	17	18	19	20	
																				X/
21	22	23	24	25	26	27	28	29	30	31	32	33	34	35	36	37	38	39	40	X/O
																				%

1	2	3	4	5	6	7	8	9	10	11	12	13	14	15	16	17	18	19	20	
																				X/
21	22	23	24	25	26	27	28	29	30	31	32	33	34	35	36	37	38	39	40	X/O
																				%

1	2	3	4	5	6	7	8	9	10	11	12	13	14	15	16	17	18	19	20	
																				X/
21	22	23	24	25	26	27	28	29	30	31	32	33	34	35	36	37	38	39	40	X/O
																				%

KEY: X=CORRECT AND REINFORCED /=CORRECT BUT NOT REINFORCED 0=INCORRECT

GRAND TOTAL X/______

X/O______

%______

Figure 6. Score Sheet (Reprinted with permission from Behavioral Sciences Institute, Monterey, California, copyright, 1971).

Example:

			45 sec.						83 sec.										
1	2	3	4	5	6	7	8	9	10	11	12	13	14	15	16	17	18	19	20
X	X	X	0	X	X	X	X	X	0										

Diagram 4

In this example the client spoke for forty-five seconds and then emitted a stuttered word (box 4). The client then spoke for another eighty-three seconds and emitted another stuttered word (box 10). Hence, the rate was two stuttered words in 128 seconds or approximately 1 SW/M.

SUMMARY

This chapter has been devoted to describing the mechanics of operant or programmed therapy for people who stutter. There are important skills which are vital to the operation of an operant therapy program: counting stuttered words and total words, timing, charting and scoring. The basic equipment required is a counter and a stopwatch. It is also helpful to have certain recording and scoring forms.

CHAPTER III

EVALUATION

A STANDARD INTERVIEW PROCEDURE

WE DEVELOPED TWO INTERVIEW PROTOCOLS, one for adults and one for children. The purposes of these were to provide clinicians with a format for interviewing and to explore the effects of various speaking activities on the rate of stuttering. We hypothesized that the findings from these interviews would provide information which would be helpful to us in selecting clients and designing appropriate therapy programs. We also used them as pre- and post-measures of the effects of our therapy programs. They require approximately forty minutes to administer and yield approximately twenty minutes of talking time by the person who stutters. The administration and scoring are relatively easy. The interview requires only a few materials.

There are different speech activities ranging from counting to conversation. The parts are individually timed and analyzed. Provision is made for topographical analysis of the stuttering behavior. The results are expressed in stuttering rate, verbal output rate, a list of various forms of stuttering behaviors, and an overall severity measure.

The client selection number we have used is a rate of 3 SW/M or more and/or a severity rating of 1 or more. The clinician should tape record the entire interview to permit a recheck of various items.

SI, Form A., Pre-School, Primary

The first is the Pre-School/Primary Form of the Stuttering Interview (SI) which requires the following material:

1. Reading material at the child's reading level
2. 15-20 pictures
3. 2 puppets

STUTTERING INTERVIEW (SI)
FORM A
Pre-School Primary

Name: ______________________ Age: __________ Sex: __________

Tester: __________________ Total: SW/M __________ Severity: 0 1 2 3 (circle one)

Date: __________________ Reliability: __________%

Time Sec.	Number of Stuttered Words (SW)		
		A.	**Automatic:** 1. "Count from 1-20" (less for young children) 2. "Say alphabet", "days of week", "months of year" 3. "Sing a Song" (tester may suggest one) 4. "Tell a nursery rhyme" or "poem" (tester may suggest one
		B.	**Echoic:** (say after tester one at a time) 5. car man paper yesterday happiness competition see that. He can go. The cat jumped up. Mother and he will go to the store.
		C.	**Read:** (material at or below child's reading level) 6. "Read aloud". (100 words or 1 minute)

		D.	**Pictures:**
			7. Name 10 pictures
		E.	**Speak Alone:** (tester leaves room)
			8. "Talk about anything" (1 minute)
		F.	**Speak with puppet:**
			9. Have two puppets talk to each other (1 minute)
		G.	**Monologue:**
			10. Talk about recent movie or trip or T.V. show (1 minute)
		H.	**Commands:** (tester demonstrates)
			11. Give tester five commands which he or she does
		I.	**Talk and Gesture:** (tester demonstrates)
			12. Tell and show how to get a drink, or put on clothing, or hit a ball.

SI-A-2

Time Sec.	Number of Stuttered Words (SW)		
		J.	**Competition:** (tester says different items simultaneously)
			13. "Say nursery rhyme" or "pledge of allegiance" (give two trials)
		K.	**Phonemic difficulty:** (say after tester one at a time)
			14. "Say these words": (Give two trials, if necessary) aluminum cinnamon vinegar constitutional multisyllabic preservation spaghetti
		L.	**Speed:**
			15. "Name as many things in the room as you can while I count to ten, hurry" or, "Tell me what you did today as fast as you can, hurry", (give two trials)
		M.	**Talk and draw:** (tester demonstrates)
			16. "Draw something and tell about it as you draw it. I will close my eyes and try to guess what it is from your talking".

		N.
		Questions:
		17. "What does your father do? What does your mother do? Do you have any brothers or sisters? Tell me about them. Do you have any pets? Tell me about them."
		18. "Ask me five questions".
		O.
		Telephone:
		19. Have conversation on toy telephone (1 minute).
		P.
		Conversation:
		20. Conversation. "You have done a fine job. Now let's just talk". (Engage in conversation about any topic. 3 minutes).
		Q.
		Observation in a Natural Setting:
		21. Observe the child in conversation with someone other than tester in a setting other than the test room (3 minutes). Location__________ Other person __________
		TOTAL

$\frac{\text{Total SW}}{\text{Total Time in minutes}}$ = ________, = ________ SW/M

SI-AB-3

SUMMARY:

1. Reliability = $\frac{\text{\# SW Counted by Observer 1}}{\text{\# SW Counted by Observer 2}}$ x 100 = ________________% (agreement)

2. Item, Mode, and Rate:	3. Type Classification (count each or simply check if present):				
	Whole Word W/W	Part Word P/W	Prolongation P	Struggle S	Other Oth
C/C Reading: Total SW_______ WR_______/ Time_______ = SW/M_______ WR/M_______					
G/F Monologue: Total SW_______ WS_______/ Time_______ = SW/M_______ WS/M_______					
P/H Conversation: Total SW_______ WS_______/ Time_______ = SW/M_______ WS/M_______					
Total Types					
% Types					

$\frac{\text{\# one type}}{\text{\# total types}}$ x 100 =

* Other (describe)____

4. Severity	0	1	2	3
SW/M	0–.5	.6–5	6–10	11+
WS/M or WR/M	100+	90–99	70–89	69–
Type	W/W	PW	P or Other	S

Scale		Severity
0–.4	normal	0
.5–1	mild	1
1.1–2	moderate	2
2.1–3	severe	3

Total Score = ______ / 3 = ______ Scale

INSTRUCTIONS:

1. Tape record entire SI (except Item Q/J). Time only client's talking or reading time.
2. Do word count and type analysis (from tape recording).
3. Omit items child cannot perform.
4. Count stuttered words as whole word repetitions, part-word repetitions, prolongations, and struggle. Count each stuttered word only once.
5. In type classification if two or more types of stuttering occur on one word count or classify the more or most severe type.
6. Do reliability rating with one other person from tape recorder in reading or in monologue if person is a non-reader.
7. Compute severity rating by selecting the highest stuttering rate from the three modes, the lowest speaking or reading rate from the three modes, and the type score which is derived from the occurrence of various forms of stuttering.
8. May give only items: C/C Reading, G/F Monologue and P/H Conversation as a Screening Test.

Figure 7. Stuttering Interview (SI) form A, pre-school, primary (Reprinted with permission from Behavioral Sciences Institute, Monterey, California, copyright, 1971).

4. Paper and crayons or pencils for drawing
5. Toy telephone (or a real one)

The form is shown in Figure 7. The instructions for administration and scoring are shown on page three of the interview.

The final part of the interview is a summary page which permits a deeper analysis of the client's stuttering behavior in three critical tasks: reading, monologue and conversation. These samples are analyzed for stuttering rate, word output rate and topography. One may either simply indicate the presence of a certain type of stuttering or its actual total frequency and percentage of relative frequency of occurrence may be computed. This information is then used to compute a severity statement, as per the instructions at the bottom of the page. Severity is ranked from 0, normal speaking; to 3, severe stuttering.

Example

Client S.T. has a stuttering rate of 5.7 SW/M, a word rate of 75 WR/M and there are part-word repetitions, whole word repetitions and prolongations in his stuttering. He is scored 2 points for 5.7 SW/M, 2 points for 75 WR/M and 2 points for having prolongations, a total of 6 points. The 6 is then divided by 3 which yields a scale score of 2. This score reads out on the severity scale to be a severity rating of 2.0 or moderate.

Try these: (The answers will follow.)

A. Client M.F. has a SW/M of 17.4, WS/M of 90, and struggle behavior, His severity rating is . . . .
B. Client T.S. has a SW/M of .5, WS/M of 125, and whole word repetitions. Her severity rating is . . . .

A. Severity is 3 (severe stutterer).
B. Severity is 0 (normal speaker).

The severity rating may have prognostic value and may be helpful to the clinician to decide priorities.

A summary of the data collected on sixteen male and female clients ranging in age from five to twelve is shown in Table IV.

The results indicate that stuttering rate varied as a function of the speaking task. As can be seen by the large standard devia-

TABLE IV

RESULTS OF STUTTERING INTERVIEW (SI), FORM A, FOR 16 MALE AND FEMALE CLIENTS

Item	Stuttered Words per Minute Mean	S.D.	Rank (From Least Stuttering 1 to Most Stuttering 17)
A 1-4 Automatic	2.1	2.9	2
B 5 Echoic	2.9	3.8	3
C 6 Read	5.5	5.6	10
D 7 Name pictures	1.0	2.0	1
E 8 Speak alone	4.3	4.0	6
F 9 Speak with puppet	5.4	7.6	9
G 10 Monologue	8.2	8.2	16
H 11 Commands	6.6	8.1	14.5
I 12 Talk and gesture	6.6	6.7	14.5
J 13 Competition	5.9	4.6	11
K 14 Phonemic complexity	4.0	4.5	4
L 15 Speed	4.5	7.5	7
M 16 Talk and draw	4.7	5.8	8
N 17 Questions examiner	12.4	15.1	17
18 Questions client	6.3	5.9	12
O 19 Telephone	4.1	3.8	5
P 20 Conversation	6.4	4.0	13
Total SW/M	5.3	2.6	
Total talking time	18.1	5.8	
Total age	8.3	2.0	

tions there was much variation from client to client. The group means do give some information about the relative difficulty of different speaking situations. The situation which evoked the most stuttering was questioning by the tester. The least stuttering evoking situation was naming pictures, usually one word utterances. It was predicted that commands, and talking and gesturing, would evoke little stuttering, but these items turned out to be highly stuttering evoking. Another surprise was that phonemic complexity was one of the lowest ranked. This may have been because the words were repeated, similar to the echoic section. If these words had been read or spontaneously generated by the children, they may have evoked more stuttering. Reading was ranked in the median position. Some children experienced more difficulty in reading than in conversation and vice-versa.

Silverman (1971a; 1971b; 1971c) reported that normal disfluency frequency of her four normal speaking preschool subjects was the function of types of speaking (more in social than in egocentric), and location of speaking event (more disfluency at home than at school or in an interview at school).

Because we wanted the clinician to look at the child in a speaking situation other than in the clinic or clinic room, we recently added Item Q. to the interview after collecting data on all the other items. We do not have data on this item at this time. We eliminated a picture story telling item because it was so similar to monologue. An interruption item was also eliminated because it was too difficult to administer in a standard fashion.

The sequence for individual children suggests directions that therapy approaches might take. For example, the child who read fluently could start a program with reading. This procedure would be similar to that employed by Egolf, et al. (1972) in which they analyzed parent-child interaction and determined therapy procedures from this analysis.

SI, Form B., Upper Elementary, Junior High, Senior High, Adult

The second form is the Upper Elementary, Junior High, Senior High and Adult version of the Stuttering Interview (SI). It requires the following materials and equipment:

1. Magazine with pictures
2. Reading material (Amplier Passage from Fairbanks, 1960)
3. Real telephone

The form is shown in Figure 8. The instructions for administration and scoring are the same as for SI, Form A.

The data for twenty male clients ranging in age from thirteen to forty-three are shown in Table V.

The results indicate that stuttering rate varied as a function of the different speaking situations. There was much individual variation. The situation which evoked the least amount of stuttering was talking alone. The most stuttering was produced in the speaking situation where the client had to ask the clinician some questions. Reading evoked more stuttering than conversation or monologue. The echoic, monologue and conversation items did not differ greatly from each other.

STUTTERING INTERVIEW (SI)
FORM B

Upper Elementary   Junior High   Senior High   Adult

Name: ______________________ Age: ________ Sex: ________

Tester: ______________ Total: SW/M ____________ Severity: 0 1 2 3 (circle one)

Date: ______________ Reliability: ____________ %

Time Sec.	Number of Stuttered Words	
		A.
		B.
		C.

A. Automatic:

1. "Count to 20".
2. "Say alphabet" or "days of week" or "months of year".
3. "Say a poem" or "the pledge of allegiance"
4. "Sing a song".

B. Echoic: (say after tester one at a time)

5. car man Ann goodbye paper interest stuttering amphibians cooperation specialization organizational representational constitutional some day the house into the car I can't find her. It's a good idea Yesterday it rained for hours.

C. Read: ("Amplifier" Passage[1] with 300 words or comparable passage)

6. "Read aloud"

			D. **Pictures:** (any magazine)
			7. Name 10 pictures.
			E. **Speak alone:** (tester leaves room)
			8. "Talk about anything" (1 minute).
			F. **Monologue:**
			9. "Tell me about recent T.V. program or movie you saw" (1 minute).
			G. **Questions:**
			10. "What is your name? Where do you work or attend school? What exactly do you do there? What does your father/husband do? What does your mother/wife do? How many are in your family? Tell me about them".
			11. "Ask me five questions".
			H. **Conversation:** (tester may take case history)
			12. Tester engages in conversation with person about his speech; history of the problem, previous therapy, therapy goals, difficult speaking situations, other problems (3 minutes).

SI-B-2

Time Sec.	Number of Stuttered Words	
		I.
		J.
		Total

Telephone:

13. Place three calls.
    Call airlines or bus lines. "What time does the ______ from ______ arrive.
    Call a friend or relative and chat.
    Answer a classified ad or call a store about a desired item. (total time 1 minute).

Observation in a natural setting:

14. Observe the person in conversation with someone other than the tester in a setting other than the test room. (3 minutes)
    Location ____________ Other person ______________________

$$\frac{\text{Total SW}}{\text{Total Time in minutes}} = \_\_\_\_\_\_\_\_, = \_\_\_\_\_\_\_\_ \text{ SW/M}$$

[1] Fairbanks, G. Voice and Articulation, New York: Harper Brothers, 1960, p. 114

NOTES:

Figure 8. Stuttering Interview (SI) form B, upper elementary, junior high, senior high, adult (Reprinted with permission from Behavioral Sciences Institute, Monterey, California, copyright, 1971).

TABLE V

RESULTS OF STUTTERING INTERVIEW (SI), FORM B, FOR 20 MALE CLIENTS

Item			Stuttered Words per Minute Mean	S.D.	Rank (From Least Stuttering 1 to Most Stuttering 11)
A	1-4	Automatic	6.1	8.1	2
B	5	Echoic	8.8	6.8	8
C	6	Read	10.5	9.8	9
D	7	Pictures	8.1	6.0	5
E	8	Speak alone	5.5	4.5	1
F	9	Monologue	8.6	6.6	7
G	10	Questions examiner	7.7	5.3	3
	11	Questions client	18.3	13.5	11
H	12	Conversation	8.6	6.1	6
I	13	Telephone	10.6	5.8	10
J	14	Conversation/strangers	8.0	7.3	4
Total SW/M			9.2	3.4	
Total talking time			20.9	11.6	
Total age			23.2	8.8	

The results of the older clients (thirteen years of age and older) compared to the younger clients (twelve years of age and younger) indicated a higher rate of stuttering for the older group. This is to be expected as age is generally related to stuttering severity (Luper and Mulder, 1964). The telephone which ranked high for adults was ranked relatively low for children. The adults had more difficulty asking questions whereas the children demonstrated more difficulty answering questions. Automatic speech was ranked similarly (second least stuttering evoking) for both children and adults, although adults stuttered more than children during automatic speaking activities.

The interview gives the clinician an opportunity to collect and observe a sample of the client's speech in a wide variety of speaking experiences. The clinician can also get some indication about the relative difficulty of the various situations and the stability across situations. We have found the SI a helpful tool to evoke, measure, and evaluate stuttering behavior; to make the decision as to whether or not a client needs fluency training, and to use as a pre- and post-measure of the effects of therapy.

BASE RATE OR CRITERION TEST

After we have decided that the client needs fluency training we begin our second sampling process. This process is referred to as Base Rate or, in program terminology, Criterion Test. It is a Base Rate in that it is a measure of the client's stuttering behavior pre-therapy (a base) and it is important that we get a consistent, reliable rate of stuttering before starting modification. It is a Criterion Test, in the program sense, in that we need a measure of the target behavior (fluency) before the therapy program and after it so that we may determine the effects of our program and whether or not to move a client ahead in the program.

The test is characterized by having the client read, engage in monologue and converse with the clinician. During this test the clinician avoids any special reaction to the client's stuttering. This permits the client to adapt to the situation. The test is to obtain a sample of the client's *normal* stuttering behavior, which provides the clinician with a reference point against which later changes can be compared. The clinician counts stuttered words, total words, and times the talking of the client. This information is charted and recorded on the data sheet.

In the clinic or therapy setting, we commonly ask the client to read for five minutes, monologue for five minutes and converse with us for five minutes. We usually only do this once. However, this process may be repeated to determine the stability of the rate of stuttering. It is highly recommended by various authorities (Goldiamond, 1965; Holland and Skinner, 1961; Sidman, 1962; Bandura, 1969; Martin and Siegel, 1966a) that we continue Base Rate measures until the client's rate stabilizes.

The definition of stabilization varies both with the client and the mode of verbal behavior. Some clients demonstrate more stability of response rate than others. Reading tends to be more stable than conversation. Goldiamond (1965) found that stability was not difficult to obtain. Our own experience has been the same. For a specific measure of stabilization we refer the reader to Martin and Siegel (1966b). The higher the rate of stuttering, the more variability is observed and acceptable. Commonly, we compare the Base Rate or Criterion Test measure with that ob-

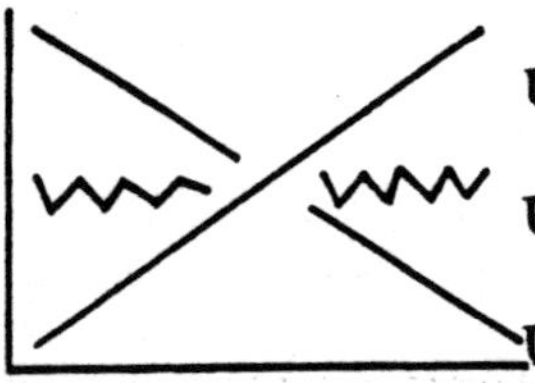

Diagram 5

tained in reading, monologue and conversation during the SI. Generally, we find the rates similar enough to permit us to move ahead into therapy with confidence that we have an accurate, stable measure of the person's stuttering behavior.

Only if we observe unusual increase or decrease in stuttering response rate do we collect additional Base Rates. We do so until the rate reaches an asymptote, disappears, or continues to show reasonable variation around a mean (± 1 SW/M per each 5 SW/M, e.g. with a mean of 15 SW/M, permit ± 3 SW/M variation, after Martin and Siegel).

Our early fear that clients would adapt to the Base Rate situation and become fluent before we could start our programs has not been supported by our experience. Adaptation is not a problem. The common study of adaptation reported in the literature (Johnson, 1955) has been of successive readings of the same material. We are constantly varying both read and spoken material and have not seen extensive adaptation.

Base Rate measures are commonly taken in the therapy setting. However, it is important to know the client's Base Rate of stuttering in other environments. We assume that the rate in the therapy setting is comparable to the rate in other settings, but we do not have much data on this. What little data we do have suggest that the rate is comparable, but further verification is necessary before we can be sure. We are in the process of collecting this information through the use of a portable, wireless microphone which is worn by our clients. If possible, the clinician should get samples of the client's rate of stuttering in the classroom, and/or work, and/or home setting (this is now part of the SI procedure just discussed). If the client has access to a tape recorder, several periods of reading, monologue and conversation at home or at work can be recorded. These can then be analyzed by the clinician to determine the client's Base Rate in those settings. We have done this on several clients and the results were that the rates were stable and quite similar to what we observed in the clinic.

Another possibility is to train the clients to count their own stuttered words and let them take their own count samples in a wide variety of normal settings. This procedure does have the disadvantage of making the client aware of stuttering, which in itself could affect the frequency of occurrence of stuttering.

The basic elements of a Base Rate or Criterion Test sample are counting and timing, with no special instructions or consequences by the clinician. This rate measure is taken before a program is started and after different therapy phases. The difference among these various Base Rates is a measure of the effectiveness of the therapy program. We do not yet know the optimum length of the Base Rate or Criterion Test, or which speaking situations are the most representative of stuttering. We have assumed that five minutes is enough of a time sample, and that reading, monologue and conversation are appropriate speaking situations. These procedures have been functional, but we need research to validate them.

SUMMARY

This chapter discussed two procedures for collecting and analyzing samples of client's speech. The Stuttering Interview (SI) is to help the clinician make the initial decision about whether or not the person is a candidate for fluency training. It may also be used for post-testing purposes after therapy.

The Base Rate or Criterion Test is to provide a pre-therapy measure and a post-therapy measure to determine the effects of therapy and/or the need for further fluency training.

CHAPTER IV

PROGRAMMING

DEFINITION AND DESCRIPTION OF PROGRAMS

A PROGRAM IS DEFINED as a series of steps which provide a learning experience for the learner by going through small, successive approximations of the desired end-goal behavior until the desired end-goal behavior is attained.

Programs usually start with behaviors already within the learner's repertoire and gradually lead to the final behavior. In other words, programs usually start with easy steps and end with hard steps. Each step is clearly defined in terms of stimulus, response and consequence. The steps are so designed that the learner receives continual, immediate feedback concerning the adequacy of the response. Step size, sequence and relationship to the final desired behavior are carefully considered.

The programmer selects the content of the program and arranges it in a sequence which will provide for a maximum of success and a minimum of failure in a reasonable amount of time. The steps in the program must relate to and eventually culminate in the end-goal behavior. Programs are usually first put in written form, then tested on learners and revised on the basis of the learners' performance.

There are many different formats and rules for program writing and evaluation (Pipe, 1966; Silverman, 1971; Mager, 1962; Cram, 1961; Edling, 1969; Espich and Williams, 1967; Markle, 1964). On the following pages we would like to expand on the above points of programming and show how they pertain to programs for fluency training.

BEHAVIORAL OBJECTIVES

The programmer starts by defining the last step in the program or the desired terminal behavior, the target for the program.

This objective or objectives must be very clearly defined and measurable (Mager, 1962). It must state who, what, when, where, and how well the behavior is to be performed.

The desired target behavior for all people who stutter is:

> Speak fluently to all people in all situations in a wide variety of speaking situations permanently.

To achieve this end we have broken that major behavioral objective down into some sub-objectives such as:

> Read fluently at 0 SW/M to an audience of one (the clinician) for five minutes in the clinic therapy room.

and,

> Speak fluently at 0 SW/M to ten different people in stores, restaurants, and other public places for a total of five minutes.

and,

> Speak fluently at 0 SW/M during repeated yearly Criterion Tests for two years.

These behavioral objectives have been written and are to be found in the program format itself in Chapter V which contains illustrations of actual programs. The behavioral objectives are listed as steps and tests throughout the programs. Their statement and measurement provide the program core.

SELECTING CONTENT

The selection of a content or repertoire of behaviors to put into a program for fluency training is important. We might view the three aspects of stuttering; speech, anxiety and attitude and prepare programs for each of these. Actually this has already been done in a limited manner (Brutten and Shoemaker, 1967; Gray, 1969; Shames, 1970; Ryan, 1970; Haroldson, Martin and Starr, 1968; Martin and Haroldson, 1970).

The focus of this book is on speech. The selection of content of speech fluency programs presents a number of choices. The program could train for identification of stuttering, pullouts, cancellations (Van Riper, 1963) or it could train for easy talking (Williams, 1971) or it could train for fluency through any means, such as the metronome (Brady, 1969; Meyer and Comley, 1969), or masking (Perkins and Curlee, 1969). The speech fluency programs in this book teach several of these behaviors as will be seen in Chapter V.

One final point is that a content should be selected which will have an impact on the target behavior. The data suggest that appropriate content for a program to help people who stutter should focus on speech fluency. A program to help a person who stutters to recite the various theories of stuttering may have little or no impact on the person's ability to speak fluently. Anxiety reduction procedures may not eliminate stuttering speech (Gray, 1969). Appropriate selection of content is critical to program construction lest much time and energy be spent on teaching skills and behaviors which are unrelated to the target behavior.

STEP SEQUENCE AND SIZE

Once the behaviors are described and listed it becomes important to list them in an appropriate sequence. In my first effort at programming (Ryan, 1964) I listed three levels of cancellation: 1) repeat the stuttered word, 2) repeat it and prolong the vowel and 3) repeat it and prolong the initial consonant. This is an illustration of the sequencing of tasks. They need to be in a reasonable, logical order and culminate in the final target behavior. Often a sequence that looks good on paper will not be supported by client performance. Our telephone programs have been especially difficult for this reason. Is answering the telephone easier or harder than calling someone and asking a question? We have found much individual variation in this and consequently partly solved the problem by putting the telephone program sequence toward the end of the total therapy program.

Step size is also critical. If steps are too large, clients fail and are frustrated. If they are too small, clients become bored or the program simply takes too long.

INSTRUCTIONS

Most clinicians are used to giving a lot of instructions to their clients. Operant therapy is different. Most operant programs rely heavily on the client's performance and the clinician's evaluation of the performance. The clinician gives minimal instructions and is very careful to reinforce these instructions accurately. Instructions are often re-administered when the person fails a step or misses a stuttered word. They serve as reinforcers, punishers, and cues for better responses, but they are commonly held to a minimum and are extremely specific. Instructions are important stimuli to guide and evoke desired behaviors. They should be used carefully. Good programs provide for a high rate of client responding and a low rate of clinician instruction.

CRITERION

The term *criterion* usually means a standard. In this usage it means the level of performance by the client. We commonly use zero stuttered words per minute (0 SW/M) for circumscribed time periods (five minutes). Criterion levels tell how well the client must perform on each step before going to the next.

Another kind of criterion is accuracy of performance as measured by the per cent of correct responses out of total responses. If out of ten stuttered words the client was able to cancel eight of them, this would yield 80 per cent accuracy. We commonly use 90 per cent. However, if the total stuttering rate is low (under ten), we use another system.

Another kind of criterion is to set the number of responses for which a certain level of performance is to be maintained. We commonly use ten consecutive correct responses (fluent sentences for example).

CONSEQUENCES

Programs should be designed so that appropriate consequences occur immediately after each response has been emitted. If the response is undesirable, then the consequence should be a negative one (a stuttered word is followed by the clinician saying "no," or nothing. If the response is a desired one, then the consequence should be a positive one (a fluent word is followed by the clinician saying, "good"). The consequences are commonly called positive reinforcers or punishers depending on the role they play. It is important to decide which events are reinforcers and which are punishers. Attention by the clinician may be either a positive reinforcer or a punisher. This can be determined by observing the effect it has on the client's behavior. If asked, some clients will tell what events they like or do not like.

In most of our programs we have used social reinforcement (saying, "right, good job, good") and punishers like "no, say it again," or saying nothing. For most clients, both children and adults, these reinforcers and punishers coupled with small-step programs have been sufficient to produce the desired changes.

With some negative, disturbed or very young children we have had to use other forms of reinforcement. Tangible rewards like candy, toys, money and games are very helpful with children who do not want to go to therapy, or who do not want to work on their speech. These rewards do tend to have excellent motivational value to get the child to attend and respond, but are not necessary for every child. They should be paired with social reinforcement. The common arrangement is to use points or tokens (beans, or poker chips, or toothpicks, or marks on a paper, etc.) which are given immediately to the child for each correct response and accompanied by *good* or *right*. These points or tokens may be totaled at the end of a session or a week or a month and turned in for some specified tangible reward like candy, etc. The token system permits immediate feedback and yet does not have the distracting value that giving the real item to the child might have at that moment. We have also removed tokens or points for inaccurate responses. This can be very powerful. To avoid satiation, it is important to set the exchange rate quite high so that not more than one small toy or bit of candy or five cents is earned in any one session. Preferably these additional reinforcers should be faded out toward the end of a program so that the client will be working for social reinforcement only. This is much more common in the world and makes transfer more likely. Token systems are discussed extensively by Ayllon and Azrin (1968).

We have had good success with children by asking them what they would like as a reinforcer. For some it has been special privileges, for others some favorite food, school supplies, and so on. After questioning the child, we list the rewards on paper so that the child knows the value of the points being earned. For high school students it may be a grade in *speech class,* or some spending money, or a ticket to a social or athletic event, or released time from speech therapy.

One interesting reinforcer is to show the client the chart to watch the rate decrease during a program. For many clients this is very reinforcing. For other clients released time from therapy has been reinforcing. Points will earn minutes off from therapy. A client may *buy* a whole session off, eventually. For extremely negative clients the clinician may have to attach positive consequences to pre-therapy behaviors such as attendance, cooperation in the setting, paying attention, talking during therapy, etc.

SCHEDULES OF REINFORCEMENT

The scheduling of the reinforcement is a critical variable and may well determine the long-term effects of therapy. A continuous schedule of reinforcing each and every response is very good to start out with because it helps the client to perform well soon, but it should be changed to intermittent at some point in the program to provide for maintenance of the response rate.

We have used a schedule which starts out high with 100 per cent reinforcement which then fades to 50 per cent (every other correct response, or every two correct responses, or any half out of a set number of correct responses) and finally to 10 per cent (every ten correct responses out of one hundred).

BRANCHING AND PLACEMENT

Two somewhat sophisticated concepts of programming are branching and placement. Branching refers to a process which allows for additional training when a client fails a step. The simplest form of branching is reinstruction. We tell the client again what is to be done. One may write a program which has no failure, but it is apt to be very long and bore all but the worst client. Our programs generally are easy for most clients, but there are some who fail and need additional procedures. Failure is defined as three sessions or forty minutes on a step without passing. There are branches, or steps between steps which can be helpful. For a client who cannot do a cancellation step even after several sessions we have a branch step in which the clinician models the desired cancellation behavior for the client. Usually with branch step procedures the client can return to the main program step and continue through the program. We also have an *open* branch step (branch step 245) which requires the clinician to problem solve the situation. It is possible that some subtle, highly individualized problem is the reason why the client cannot pass the regular step. For example, the client who has special, extreme, specific word fears such as fear of words starting with /s/ might be unable to pass a step because of that factor. The perceptive clinician then might institute a special branch step procedure to give the client special practice on /s/ words. There may be debilitating personal or family problems which are so depressing that the client cannot pass any steps on any program. These must be solved by special branching procedures by the perceptive clinician including taking the client off the program until other problems are solved.

Placement is the process whereby a client can move ahead, skip steps and generally complete a program ahead of schedule. We occasionally find someone who does not stutter when reading. This client would be placed on the next procedure (monologue) beyond reading. We do not have much placement in the fluency programs except for this kind of gross moving ahead or elimination of phases when a client demonstrates special ability during a Criterion Test.

PROGRAM FORMAT

It is necessary to have a format in which to write out the program steps and all the necessary additional statements such as criterion, responses, etc. Such a format was developed by Gray and reported by Gray and Fygetakis (1968). The format with examples is shown in Figure 9.

The stimulus column lists the activities of the clinician. These are usually some form of instruction, modeling, or other stimulus presentation such as holding up a picture. In addition, of course, the clinician is also reinforcing, counting and timing during each session.

Stimulus	Response	Schedule (Sch)	Criterion (C)	Branch Index (BI)
Instructions, models and/or materials What the clinician says and does before the client responds	Description of the response desired from the client	How often to provide a reinforcer	The per cent of correct responses, or number of successively correct responses, or stuttering rate per time	The number of the step to go to, if there is failure
Examples:	*Examples:*	*Examples:*	*Examples:*	*Examples:*
"Speak slowly and fluently" "Say, house" a picture	1 fluent word 1 fluent sentence fluent conversation	100 per cent or 50 per cent or 10 per cent of the time after correct responses	90 per cent correct, or 10 correct responses in a row, or .5 stuttered words a minute for 5 minutes	BI 27 or BI 28 or 245

Figure 9. Program Format (Gray).

The response column describes the desired response of the client in each step. The response is gradually expanded in each successive step.

The schedule or "sch" column indicates the schedule of reinforcement or when to give the client a reward or punisher (say "good," give a token, or say "no"). A 100 means that every correct response is reinforced, 50 means that every other correct response is reinforced and 10 means that every tenth response is reinforced. These latter two reinforcement schedules should be on an intermittent basis, i.e. out of twenty responses, ten should be reinforced, but not necessarily every other one. Out of twenty responses, two should be reinforced, but not necessarily the tenth and the twentieth. For intermittent reinforcement to be truly effective, it should be given on a random basis varying around a mean.

The criterion or "C" column tells about the adequacy of a response which is listed as a level of per cent correct, or number of consecutively correct responses, or rate of stuttering per circumscribed time period. A client must meet the criterion in one session. If not completed, the step is started over at the beginning of the next session.

The Branch Index or BI column lists the number of the branch step procedure to be followed in the event of failure. The branch index steps themselves are usually listed somewhere else.

PROGRAM PHASES

There are five program phases; response evaluation, response evocation, establishment, transfer, and maintenance.

Response Evaluation Phase

This phase is usually not a formal part of the program proper. It refers to a skill which the clinician must bring to the program. In the case of fluency programs it refers to the skill of the clinician in identifying and counting stuttered words and fluent words. The clinician must possess this skill or the programs cannot be run successfully. Most programmed therapy procedures assume that speech clinicians' professional training has provided them with this skill. However, unfortunately, such is not the case. Very few university training programs offer training in counting stuttered words. Clinicians must attend special workshops or train themselves (see Ryan and Van Kirk, 1973, in bibliography).

Response Evocation Phase

This phase refers to getting that first response in the program. It is important that the client be able to get past the first step. Most of the fluency programs in this book start with simple responses so that most clients do pass the first step. Occasionally a client will need additional pre-program training. In one program, the client is asked in Step one to say only one word fluently. We have had a few clients who could not do even that simple task. It was necessary to take them to whispering that one word to help them and then they moved on to the regular step.

Establishment Phase

This phase of the program refers to having the client acquire the new response. Fortunately, in the case of stuttering, all the clients have fluency within their repertoires. Few people who stutter do so on every word. Establishment really refers to increasing the frequency of a response, fluency, which is already in the client's repertoire, rather than to teaching a new response. The establishment phase is operationally defined as that phase during which the client learns to converse fluently in the presence of the clinician in the clinic setting.

Transfer Phase

This phase of the program refers to helping the client generalize or transfer the new, increased fluency to a number of different speaking situations. The target of this phase is fluent conversational speech in a wide variety of settings.

Maintenance Phase

This refers to a program phase to continue, indefinitely, the newly established and transferred fluency.

These five program phases have evolved out of the past nine years of research. It is important at this time to examine each of these phases. In the future, research may indicate the relative importance of each and undoubtedly there will be changes in emphasis, and possibly a reduction in the amount of training and/or phases necessary to produce fluent speech which is permanent.

TESTS AND MEASUREMENT

A hallmark of the operant or programmed instructional system is its high frequency of testing. Clients are either being tested or trained continuously. Each step in a program could be viewed as mini-test. The client is given a grade or knowledge of results after each response.

The tests of a program are: 1) the pre- and post-evaluation of it in terms of producing the target behavior, 2) the length of time a program takes or in program language, its *run time* (a more critical measure may be number of responses) and finally 3) the per cent accuracy during the program. All of these measures should be made of a program so that it may be designed correctly to offer the greatest amount of improvement to the most people in the shortest amount of time.

The pre- and post-testing we use employs both the Stuttering Interview (SI) and the Criterion Test (CT). One or both of these have been given to all of our clients several times during the program usually before and after establishment, after transfer and occasionally after maintenance phases.

Our target has been normal fluent speech, hence all of our measures have been of that. It would be helpful to measure both anxiety and attitude in some format if for no reason other than to document their changes. Thus far, we have not done so. Casual observation has suggested that anxiety decreases and there is improvement in attitude.

The length of time a program takes is somewhat contingent on the criterion levels. If the criterion levels are high in terms of minutes of perfect fluency, then programs take long hours to run. If they are low, then programs run more rapidly. We have found over the past nine years that criterion levels can be lowered without reducing the efficiency of the program to the point now where our most recent programs run within ten to twenty hours of total therapy time (Ryan and Van Kirk, 1971).

The final measure of a program is its run level. Most of the programs to be described in the next chapter run at less than .5 SW/M or one could say 99.5 per cent accuracy if one assumed an average one hundred-word-per-minute-normal output per session.

CLINICIAN TASKS

The clinician must be able to carry out the procedures described in Chapters II and III. In addition, the clinician must learn to read the program format and carry out the programs as they are written. The program procedures usually include instructions, response evaluation, reinforcement of correct responses, determination of when the client reaches criterion and moving the client to the next step. Although initially this may appear to be an overwhelming task it has been our experience that the procedures themselves are not hard to learn and skill in them can be achieved with a reasonable amount of training and practice.

LENGTH AND FREQUENCY OF SESSIONS

There is no ideal length. We have worked with children and adults for as little as ten minutes a day to as much as five hours a day and have gotten results in both instances. Most of the programs now have an estimated run time so that the clinician may have some idea of how long the program will take. Under some conditions such as meeting weekly in a remote school area it may be better to work for longer periods with practice periods in between. Our common time period has been forty minutes per session for both children and adults.

Of more importance is the frequency of contact. Although no hard and fast rule can be stated, it does seem important to meet the person at least two times a week if the work is to be successful and forgetting between sessions is to be held to a minimum. Intensive, short term contacts while effective with some cases, may have drawbacks because they do not permit gradual transfer and maintenance (Prins, 1970). Ideally, both the frequency and duration of contact should be gradually decreased as shown below.

A Sample Schedule:

Weeks:	1	2	3	4	5	6	7	8	9	10	11	12	13	14	15	16
Sessions per week:	5	5	4	4	3	3	2	2	1	1	1	1	0	1	0	1
Length of session:	40	30	20	20	20	20	20	20	20	20	20	10		10		10

We have used this schedule combined with home practice periods which are tape recorded. It works very well. Peins, Lee, and McGough (1970) have reported on successful home tape recorder practice.

GROUP VS. INDIVIDUAL TRAINING

Generally the programs are designed to be run individually, but we do know of instances where they were used in group settings with the clients taking turns responding and even playing the role of clinician. We recommend individual training or at least a combination of individual and group training because the critical event in training appears to be the number of monitored responses a client can make or hours of monitored practice a client can collect. The client's response time is reduced in group settings.

SUMMARY

This chapter has been concerned with the programming process and how it applies to the design and development of fluency programs. Program development requires attention to the variables of behavioral objectives, content, instructions, consequences, reinforcement schedules and criterion levels. There are five phases to program development. Constant measurement is a necessary and important part of programming. Programs are usually run on an individual rather than a group basis.

CHAPTER V

PROGRAMS: ESTABLISHMENT

ESTABLISHMENT—The goal in this phase is fluent speech in the presence of the clinician in the clinic setting.

TYPES OF PROGRAMS

We have studied four types of operant Establishment Programs to obtain speech fluency in both children and adults: 1) a *Programmed Traditional Program* composed of cancellation, pullouts, and prolongation behaviors; 2) a *Delayed Auditory Feedback Program* which utilizes rate control and prolongations which are gradually shaped toward normal fluency; 3) a *Punishment Program* which employs the administration of an aversive consequence contingent upon each stuttered word; and 4) a *Gradual Increase in Length and Complexity of Utterance Program* which starts with single word utterances and expands to normal conversational speech. Any of these Establishment Programs will help the client develop normal fluent conversational speech and prepare him for the Transfer and Maintenance Programs. There is only one type of Transfer and Maintenance Program. This will be discussed more fully in Chapter VI. The relationship between the various Establishment Programs and the Transfer and Maintenance Programs is illustrated in Figure 10.

READING, MONOLOGUE AND CONVERSATION

The three modes of reading, monologue and conversation are used. Reading is reading aloud from material appropriate to the age level and interest of the client although we try to avoid emotional or overly humorous material with dialogue.

Monologue is the client doing all the talking. The client is in-

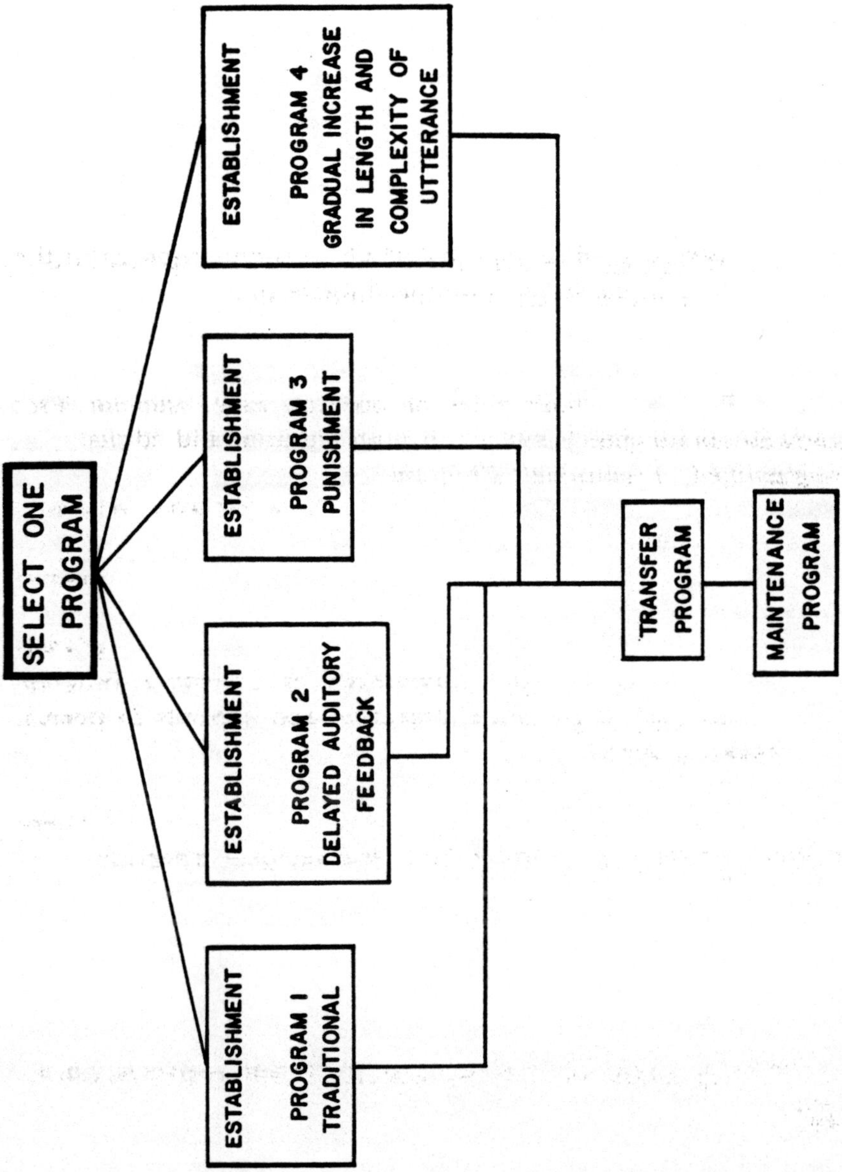

Figure 10. Relationship of establishment programs to transfer and maintenance programs.

structed to talk about any subject of interest while the clinician listens attentively. Occasionally cue cards and pictures are necessary for some clients in order to stimulate their monologue.

Conversation is talking back and forth between the clinician and the client about any topic of interest to either person or both. We try to make it a natural conversation, but this of course varies with age, interest, education and experience of the client. We try to make sure the client does most of the talking and the timing of the client's talking makes this more probable. The clinician uses both silence and simple single statements or questions to keep the conversation going.

The Establishment Programs generally start with reading, then move to monologue and terminate in conversation with review of reading and monologue during each session. The programs start with reading because this controls the client's possible circumlocution or substitution behavior and insures that the client will have something to say.

Although the programs may be run with only one of the three modes we recommend that all three be used when possible because there often is little or no transfer from one to the other. Nonreaders, of course, will not go through the reading mode. We also have run the three modes concurrently, but this presented some mechanical record keeping problems, and there appeared to be some negative transfer from one mode to another. The Transfer and Maintenance Programs employ mostly conversational speech.

OVERVIEW OF FLUENCY TRAINING

An overview of the total Fluency Training Program may be helpful before discussing each of the Establishment Programs. This is outlined in Figure 11.

The therapy process starts with referral. The client is put through a Stuttering Interview procedure (SI). If the client is a candidate for fluency training (3 SW/M or Severity of 1-3), then Criterion Test No. 1 is given. Contingent upon performance in Criterion Test No. 1, the client either goes into the reading or monologue phase or if Criterion Test No. 1 is passed, the client moves ahead to the Transfer Program. When in the Establishment Phase, the client is in one of the four Establishment

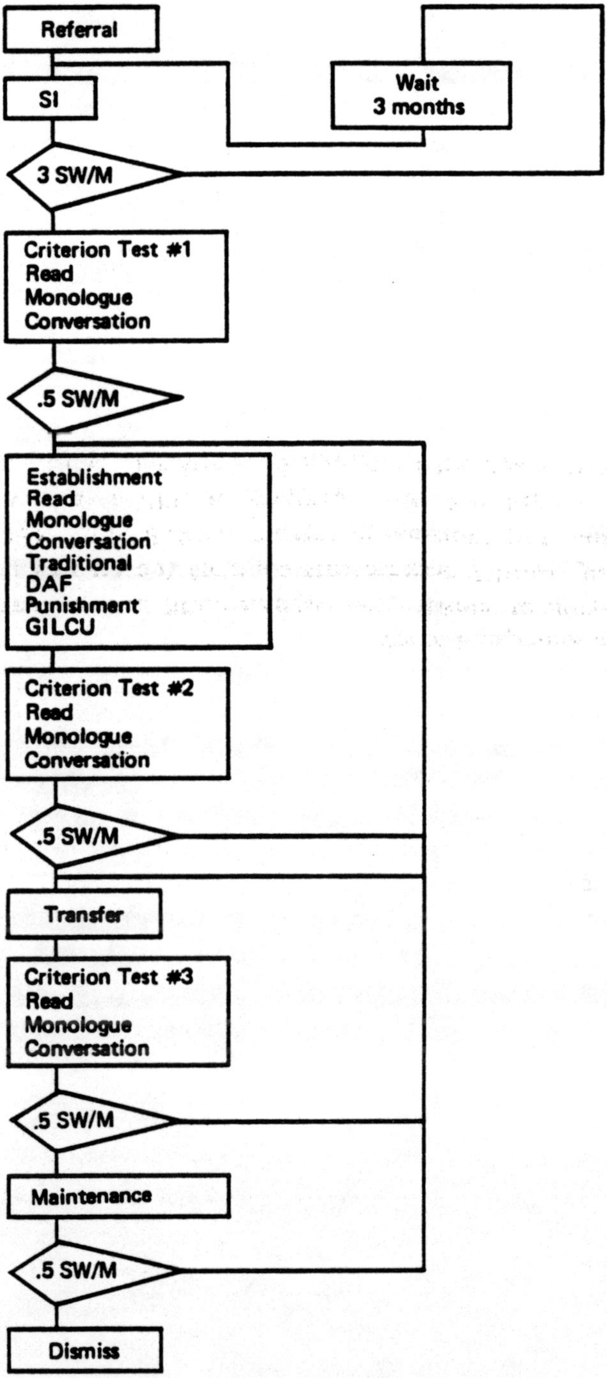

Figure 11. Outline of fluency training.

Programs. If the client demonstrates difficulty with a step for either three sessions or forty minutes, whichever comes first, the client is put on a branch sequence. When the Establishment Program is completed, the client takes Criterion Test No. 2. If the client passes (a rate of less than .5 SW/M in each of the three modes) the client goes on to the Transfer Program. If the client fails any of the modes (more than .5 SW/M) the client recycles through the Establishment Program in that mode or modes.

The client goes through the Transfer Program and on completion of that takes Criterion Test No. 3. If the client passes (less than .5 SW/M) the client goes to the Maintenance Program. If the client fails (more than .5 SW/M in any of the modes) the client is recycled through specific portions of the Transfer Program and/or Establishment Program.

The client then continues on the Maintenance Program for approximately two years. If at any time the client demonstrates a rate above .5 SW/M in any of the Maintenance Program sessions, the client is recycled for more Establishment or Transfer Program time contingent upon what the problem is.

The present programs generally run about five to ten hours in Establishment, ten to fifteen hours in Transfer and about five hours in Maintenance which is spread over two years (Ryan and Van Kirk, 1971). Individual clients, of course, may proceed faster or slower.

The clinician's basic tasks in an operant therapy program are to give instructions, count stuttered words, time the client's talking, decide when to change steps and keep a record on both the data sheet and the chart of the results of therapy and testing. Each program lists specific additional procedures for the clinician to carry out during each program which are peculiar to each program such as instructions, identifying stuttered words, modeling desired behavior, etc.

This is the overview of therapy and now we will examine the four Establishment Programs.

FOUR ESTABLISHMENT PROGRAMS

Each of the four programs will be discussed in detail. The source of the program, an outline of the program, information from the literature about the program, and run data (results) generated will be given for each program. All of the data reported on the programs were collected by the author or one of his students. We consistently used the reliability procedures described in Chapter II. We changed clinicians quarterly and it was necessary to recalibrate at the beginning of each quarter. We did this until we achieved 90 per cent agreement on the number of stuttered words in three consecutive one-minute samples of reading or monologue or conversation. All therapy sessions were tape recorded and monitored by the author for consistency of program run. Excerpts of programs on audio tape recordings of the majority of the clients reported are on file with the author.

Establishment Program 1: Programmed Traditional

This program is shown in coded form in Figure 12 and in decoded form in Figure 13. This program is so named because the basic behaviors of identification, cancellation, pullouts, prolongations and preparatory sets have long been described in the literature as part of the symptomatic therapy for stuttering (Van Riper, 1939; 1947; 1954; 1963; Sheehan, 1951; 1958; 1970; Sheehan and Voas, 1957; Eisenson, 1958; Gregory, 1968; 1969; Luper and Mulder, 1964).

The client is asked to identify stuttered words (steps 1-3) and then to learn to modify them through cancellations (steps 4-6), pullouts (steps 7 and 8) and prolongations (step 9), until the client can speak fluently (step 10). The program is first cycled through reading, then monologue and then conversation with the same ten steps being repeated in each mode for a total of thirty steps.

Should the client fail, be on one step without passing it for either three sessions or forty minutes, whichever comes first, the client is put on a branch program. The branch program for Establishment Program 1 is shown in Figure 14. The basic branch procedure is a modeling of the desired behavior by the clinician with 100 per cent reinforcement. The clinician does the cancellation, etc. first, then has the client do it. When the client passes the branch steps the client goes back to the regular program step. A

TITLE:	Programmed Traditional	NO:	1
TARGET:	Fluent Conversation in Clinic Therapy Room	R +:	Redeemable tokens and/or Social
COMMENTS:	Model and practice the behavior desired in Steps 4-9 briefly before each step	STEPS:	30

Step	*Stimulus*	*Response*	*Sch*	*C*	*BI*
	Take Criterion Test				
Series A					
1	Instruct client to read Identify	Read	100	1 minute	245
2	Instruct client to read and identify	Read and identify	100	1 minute	245
3	Instruct client to read and identify	Read and identify	100	1 minute 90%	245
4	Instruct client to read, repeat each stuttered word	Read, repeat stuttered word	100	5 minutes 90%	1
5	Instruct client to read and repeat each stuttered word in a prolonged manner	Read and repeat stuttered words in a prolonged manner	100	5 minutes 90%	3
6	Instruct client to read and repeat each stuttered word prolonging the first sound	Read and repeat stuttered words prolonging the first sound	100	5 minutes 90%	5
7	Instruct client to read and interrupt each stuttered word with a prolongation of the first sound	Read and interrupt stuttered words with a prolongation	50	5 minutes 90%	7
8	Instruct client to read and interrupt each stuttered word with a prolongation more quickly than in Step 7	Read and interrupt stuttered words with a prolongation more quickly	50	5 minutes 90%	7
9	Instruct client to read and prolong the first sound of any word he might stutter	Read and prolong any word he might stutter	50	5 minutes 90%	11
10	Instruct client to read as fluently as he can	Read fluently	10	5 minutes at 0 SW/M	13
Series B					
1-10	(Recycle same through monologue)	Monologue, etc.	Same	Same	Same
Series C					
1-10	(Recycle same through conversation)	Conversation, etc.	Same	Same	Same
	Take Criterion Test Go on to Transfer Program				

Figure 12. Program 1, Programmed Traditional.

Step	*Clinician Stimulus*	*Client Response*	*Clinician Schedule*	*Criterion*
1	"Read aloud. Each time you stutter on a word, I'll say 'there.'"	". . . . c-c-c-ar"	"there" every time client stutters	1 minute
2	"Read aloud. You and I will both signal each time you stutter on a word."	". . . . c-c-car" (and signals)	"there" every time client stutters	1 minute
3	"Read aloud and signal each time you stutter on a word." Clinician counts covertly.	". . . . c-c-car" (and signals)	(counts to himself every one)	1 minute 90% correct identification
4	"Read aloud. Repeat each stuttered word."	". . . . c-c-car, c-c-car" or "car"	"good" every time for cancellation	5 minutes 90% correct identification
5	"Read aloud and repeat each stuttered word in a prolonged manner."	". . . . c-c-car, caaaar"	"good" every time for cancellation	5 minutes 90% correct identification
6	"Read and repeat each stuttered word prolonging the first sound."	". . . . c-c-car, cccccar"	"good" every time for cancellation	5 minutes 90% correct identification
7	"Read aloud and interrupt each stuttered word with a prolongation of the first sound."	". . . . c-c-cccar"	"good" every other time for a pull-out	5 minutes 90% correct identification
8	"Read aloud and interrupt each stuttered word with a prolongation more quickly."	". . . . c-cccar"	"good" every other time for a pull-out	5 minutes 90% correct identification
9	"Read and prolong the first sound of any word you think you might stutter."	". . . . ccar"	"good" every other time for a prolongation	5 minutes 90% correct identification
10	"Read as fluently as you can."	". . . . car"	"good" for every 10 fluent sentences	5 minutes at 0 SW/M
11-30	Recycle monologue and conversation	Monologue or conversation	Same	Same

Figure 13. Program 1, Programmed Traditional, Decoded.

"245" branch step permits the clinician to problem solve the client's error.

Should the client have to recycle after failure on post-program Criterion Test No. 2, the client goes through the entire Establishment Program with a 90 per cent criterion for 2.5 minutes per step in place of the original five minutes criterion.

Failure Criterion on Branch Step is one session or 20 minutes.
245 = try anything reasonable that might help, including changing programs. C = continue in the program.

BI Step	*Stimulus*	*Response*	*Sch*	*C*	*Pass*	*Fail*
1	Instructions and clinician models each time	Repeats stuttered word after clinician	100	90% 5 min.	2	245
2	Instructions	Repeats stuttered word	100	90% 5 min.	C	1
3	Instructions and clinician models each time	Repeats stuttered word and prolongs	100	90% 5 min.	4	245
4	Instructions	Repeats stuttered word after clinician and prolongs	100	90% 5 min.	C	3
5	Instructions and clinician models each time	Repeats stuttered word and prolongs first sound after clinician	100	90% 5 min.	6	245
6	Instructions	Repeats stuttered word and prolongs first sound	100	90% 5 min.	C	5
7	Instructions and clinician models each time	Interrupts stuttered word with prolongation	100	90% 5 min.	8	245
8	Instructions	Interrupts stuttered word with prolongation	100	90% 5 min.	C	7
9	Instructions and clinician models each time	Interrupts stuttered word rapidly with prolongation	100	90% 5 min.	10	245
10	Instructions	Interrupts stuttered word rapidly with prolongation	100	90% 5 min.	C	9
11	Instructions and clinician models after client signals	Signals and prolongs possible stuttered word after clinician	100	90% 5 min.	12	10
12	Instructions	Prolongs possible stuttered word	100	90% 5 min.	C	11
13	Instructions and clinician models fluent sentence	Fluent sentence after clinician	100	0 SW/M 5 min.	14	245
14	Instructions	Fluent sentences	100	0 SW/M 5 min.	C	13

Figure 14. Branch Index, Program 1, Programmed Traditional.

This ten-step program consisted of eight steps originally (Ryan, 1964). The two additional steps (3 and 10) were added after the original work on three subjects was done. In its present form it has a minimal run time of 114 minutes. It has been a generally successful program, but the identification phase is critical. If the client does not do well in the identification steps, there will be trouble in later steps because the client must identify stuttering and do something else in each of the other steps. Haugen (1967b) found this program to be effective with an eighteen-year-old male. Ryan (1968a; 1970), Shames (1969b) and Shames, Egolf, and Rhodes (1969) reported successful use of this program with fewer steps.

One of two patterns is usually demonstrated by clients in this program. The first is a gradual decrease in stuttering rate over the different steps. This is common. The other less common pattern is an increase in stuttering rate until step nine at which time there is a decrease. The client will often increase his frequency of stuttering and decrease the size of each stuttering as a result of being reinforced for stuttering and modifying it. The duration and magnitude of the stutterings will gradually decrease until they are replaced entirely by diminutive prolongations and finally, by fluency.

The results on this program are shown in Table VI for nineteen clients ranging in age from ten to forty-three. Most of these data are for reading. For the last six clients; reading, monologue and conversation are included. This was the first program we worked with and our initial work focussed on reading. We used a number of different criterion time settings from five to forty minutes which caused the run time to be variable. The hours of time in the program refer to the client's talking time rather than hours of therapy. When the client is in reading and monologue modes the therapy time and talking time of the client are generally the same. In the conversation mode the therapy time is longer than the talking time of the client. When all three modes are included, therapy time is generally twice as long as talking time.

We have a total of 247 hours of run time on this program and the data generally indicate a decrease in stuttering rate. All clients demonstrated a decrease in stuttering rate except for Client

TABLE VI

RESULTS OF PROGRAM I, PROGRAMMED TRADITIONAL

Clients	Age	Sex	Pre Means of Stuttered Words per Minute			Hours of Talking Time in Program	Post Means of Stuttered Words per Minute		
			Reading	Monologue	Conversation		Reading	Monologue	Conversation
1. FC	14	M	11.6			20.9	1.2		
2. SW	43	M	11.9			23.0	.6		
3. DA	26	M	16.8			3.3	11.5		
4. MH	20	M	9.1			4.7	1.5		
5. TS	18	M	13.5			3.7	1.1		
6. DP	20	M	21.5			2.9	7.5		
7. CC	13	F	28.5			3.2	25.8		
8. RB	12	M	15.8			2.1	8.2		
9. JA	12	M	7.5			3.0	5.7		
10. DM	10	M	30.0			4.6	4.6		
11. CD	11	M	9.9			3.9	5.8		
12. DCo	25	M	1.8			31.0	9.8		
13. RW	20	M	3.5			20.7	.2		
14. HW	27	M	1.3	7.3		15.1	.9	1.9	
15. DL	29	M	2.1	8.8		24.1	.1	.5	
16. MT	19	M	7.8	2.9		19.8	2.8	1.3	
17. SS	14	M	4.0	24.0		20.4	.2	.9	
18. DH	20	M	14.6		8.8	22.2	2.9		5.6
19. RR	13	M	1.5	1.7	2.7	24.7	.3	1.0	.6
Mean	19.5		11.2	8.9	5.8	13.3	4.8	1.1	3.1
S.D.	8.1		8.6	8.9	4.3	10.0	6.2	.52	3.1

No. 12, DCo, who was a very severe stutterer with blocks of extreme duration (commonly more than a minute per block). An increase in stuttering rate actually was an improvement for him because his word rate also went up accordingly. His initial reading rate was 5 WR/M, whereas his final rate was 20 WR/M.

The program produced quite good fluency in some people although its early prototype ended with prolongations (Step 9) rather than normal fluency (Step 10). It put a premium on detection of stuttered words which was difficult for those people who had a high rate of stuttering. The program also did not routinely produce normal fluency although it did reduce stuttering. For these reasons we looked for other programs.

Establishment Program 2: Delayed Auditory Feedback

An outline of the Delayed Auditory Feedback Program is shown in Figure 15. The entire program including the branch index will be found in Ryan and Van Kirk (1971). This program is named after the delayed auditory feedback equipment which is an integral part of the program. The basic response of the client is prolongation and the procedure has been also referred to as a prolongation program (Ryan, 1970) or a rate-control program (Perkins, 1967; Curlee and Perkins, 1969). In its present form it has a minimal run time of 111 minutes.

The client learns first to identify stuttered words and then to read and speak with the delayed auditory feedback equipment at a slow rate prolonging each word like this: "Mmmmmmyyyyyy nnnnnnaaaaaammmmmmiiiiiissssssMmmmmmaaaaaarrrrrryyyyyy (My name is Mary)." Superarticulation may occur and is reinforced. It is important to avoid sing-song or choppy speech. The rate is gradually speeded up by decreasing the amount of delay in five steps: 250, 200, 150, 100, 50 milliseconds of delay and finally to 0 or no delay. The client is taken off the machine. The client's rate gradually speeds up until it approaches normal (more than 100 WS/M) and is stutter free, fluent. The client goes through the reading, monologue and conversation modes.

Should the client fail, be on one step without passing it for either three sessions or forty minutes, whichever comes first, the client is put on a branch program similar to that for Program 1.

Step	*Stimulus*	*Response*
1-3	Identification of stuttered words.	Identify stuttered words.
4	Instructions to read slowly. Set DAF at 250.	Read slowly in prolonged manner with DAF earphones.
5	Instructions to read slowly. Set DAF at 200.	Read slowly in prolonged manner with DAF earphones.
6	Instructions to read slowly. Set DAF at 150.	Read slowly in prolonged manner with DAF earphones.
7	Instructions to read. Set DAF at 100.	Read slowly in slightly prolonged manner with DAF earphones.
8	Instructions to read. Set DAF at 50.	Read with DAF earphones.
9	Instructions to read. Set DAF at 0.	Read with DAF earphones.
10	Instructions to read.	Read
11-30	Recycle with monologue and conversation.	Monologue or conversation.

Figure 15. Outline of Program 2, Delayed Auditory Feedback (DAF).

It is essentially based on taking the client back to a previous step with more reinforcement. When the client passes the branch steps, the client comes back to the regular program step.

Should the client have to recycle through the Establishment Program, after failing Criterion Test No. 2 in any mode, the client is recycled through every other step: 2, 4, 6, 8 and 10 as a review and given Criterion Test No. 2 again.

Occasionally a client will have to maintain a very slow rate to control the fluency. In this event the client is put through the basic program at a very low rate (less than 50 WR/M or WS/M). After completion of the entire DAF Establishment Program and the Transfer Program, at the slow rate, the client is put on a Rate Control Program (Ryan and Van Kirk, 1971) to speed the rate up to normal. However, this has seldom been necessary.

The Delayed Auditory Feedback or DAF Program is the most widely known and tested of all the operant speech fluency programs. There has been much research done on it. Soderberg (1969) did an extensive review of the work of Adamczyk (1959), Chase, Sutton and Rapin (1961), Goldiamond (1965),

Gross and Nathanson (1967), Gross and Gregory (1966), Ham and Steer (1967), Logue (1962), Lotzmann (1961), Naylor (1953), Neeley (1961), Soderberg (1959) and Yates (1963). Approximately 218 stutterers were seen in these studies of DAF and stuttering. It may be concluded from this review that: 1) continuous, amplified DAF has a consistent positive effect on the speech fluency of people who stutter, 2) short-term studies did not demonstrate as much effect, 3) the optimal amount of DAF may be different for different stutterers, 4) the persistence of good fluency after the subject is taken off the machine depends upon the length of time he was on it, 5) the intensity of the delayed signal is an important variable which has not been studied carefully enough and should be, and 6) the speech of stutterers under no DAF is different from the speech of nonstutterers under DAF. Webster, Schumacher and Lubker (1970) reported that several different DAF settings: .1, .2, .3, .4, and .5 seconds all produced positive changes in fluency, but there was no carryover.

Most of these studies were short term observations of the effects of DAF on stuttering. Goldiamond (1965) was one of the first to report on long term exposure to DAF. He used it both as an aversive consequence to stuttering behavior and as a continuous stimulus which (with instructions) resulted in slow, fluent, prolonged speech. His early work led to the development of a program for producing normal fluent speech by starting with 250 milliseconds of DAF and working down in 50 millisecond steps until the person was reading at a normal rate, free from stuttering behavior. Goldiamond's data for forty stutterers are reported for reading within a clinical-laboratory environment (Goldiamond, 1965). He offers no data about the generalization of fluency to speaking and to other speaking situations. He suggests that this occurs.

Perkins (1967) replicated Goldiamond's process, but used along with it some other clinical procedures such as counseling. His results generally support Goldiamond's findings. Recently, Curlee and Perkins (1969) reported on fifteen subjects using a program with the DAF sequence in conversational speech. As soon as the subjects achieved fluent conversation off the machine they were put into a time-out situation where the room was darkened from five to thirty seconds contingent upon each stuttering. Following attainment of fluency in these situations, the subjects were gradually exposed to more and more difficult speaking situations. The programs required an average thirty hours to complete. Curlee and Perkins suggest success although they do not offer any data on the long term effects of the program.

Gross and Nathanson (1967) and Gross and Gregory (1966) reported successful use of DAF procedures with stutterers as part of a total clinical program. Ryan (1968b) reported on the use of DAF with six people who stuttered. The six were put through long term programs in reading, monologue and conversation using the Goldiamond procedure. The within clinics effects were much like those reported by others, but transfer and maintenance of fluency were not measured. Ryan (1971) reported on the successful use of DAF with an eight-year-old child. The fluency did transfer to the child's environment. Van Kirk (1970) reported successful DAF therapy with three stutterers over fifty-five years of age. Ingham and Andrews (1971) used DAF programs with a number of their clients and were able to achieve good fluency. Van Kirk (1972) reported good results with another group of clients.

Related to the use of DAF as a mechanical device to help produce fluent speech are two other devices: the metronome and masking noise. These devices have been studied far less than DAF although they are similar in that they provide for a change in the intra-internal feedback system of the stutterer (Yates, 1969; 1970). They may be considered stimulus support or stimulus control devices. The use of rhythms, metronomes and masking noise to produce fluency is not new (Wingate, 1969), but there has been a renewed interest in these procedures couched in a behavior therapy or behavior modification framework. Cherry and Sayers (1956) report several experiments using masking and shadowing to successfully instate fluent speech. Brady (1969), Francella and Beech (1965), Beech and Francella (1968), Meyer and Mair (1963), Meyer and Comley (1969), Greenberg (1970), Andrews and Harris (1964) and Azrin et al. (1968) all reported on the beneficial effects of rhythmic, syllabic speech induced with and without a metronome. Jones and Azrin (1966) suggest increasing the length of the metronomic tone to produce more normal speech.

Yates (1969) in reviewing these procedures suggested that the metronome and masking devices might be more successful than the DAF in the long run because they could be used by the person in his natural environment. Trotter and Lesch (1967), Gruber (1971), Perkins and Curlee (1969) and Wepman and McFarland (1967) reported on experiences with portable masking devices which were turned on when the stutterer wanted to speak and turned off when he was listening. Careful measurement of these effects was not made, but subjective reports by the people using them were positive. Some of the people working with DAF have suggested the use of a portable unit, but few data have been collected on the effects of a portable DAF unit.

The basic element of the DAF Program is prolonged speech. This prolonged speech may be taught without the machine. Any number of timing devices such as a metronome, hand-held counter, stopwatch or reading slowly along with the client, etc. may be employed to teach fluent, slow, prolonged speech. However, arranging for the client to speed up gradually, without stuttering, is difficult without some form of discrete-step mechanical pacer.

The goal of this program is to develop a new response, *superfluent* prolonged speech, and then return it to normal rates with no prolongation. One early result we noticed was the super-fluent speaker, sounding almost like an automaton. To avoid this, we cut down on the instructions to prolong and permitted occasional pausing and other normal dysfluencies (see Chapter II).

The characteristic results of the DAF Program are a slight depression of stuttering rate during the identification process, which flattens out; and an immediate, sudden drop to .5 of less SW/M when the DAF is introduced. This reduction is maintained throughout the program although there are increases in SW/M when the client first comes off the machine. Goldiamond (1965) in the original work on this procedure utilized a controlled reading rate apparatus. Even without such equipment a change in reading rate will usually be noted. Occasionally, a client will continue to read relatively slowly (50-70 words read per minute or less) in the final steps. It is better to permit this slow rate than to instruct for increased rate which could induce stuttering. With continued practice and/or a special Rate Control Program, the client can and does increase the reading rate. Instructions to speak slowly and fluently should be faded early in the program.

The client comes out of this program being able to prolong, count stuttered words, articulate more precisely, and be generally fluent although the client may feel dependent upon the machine. The clinician can help the client avoid addiction to or dependency on the machine by adhering to the rules of the program and getting the client through the steps as quickly as possible.

The results of this program for twenty-eight clients ranging in age from eight to forty-five are shown in Table VII. Twenty-seven of the twenty-eight clients worked in reading, twenty-two in monologue and twenty-one in conversation. The pre- and post-measures were conducted without DAF. The effects of the DAF Program can be seen by the great reduction in stuttering rate produced by the DAF Program for most clients. We have 784 hours of run time (client talking time) on this program.

There was great variation in time which represents the different time periods used (from ten minutes to forty minutes) and criterion levels (1 SW/M to 0 SW/M) rather than the actual program time differences between the clients. The exceptionally long programs (Client #8, 104.7 hours; Client #11, 177.2 hours; and Client #14, 97.7 hours) were run to a criterion of forty-minute periods at 0 SW/M. The exceptionally rapid programs (Client #20, 2.5 hours; Client #23, 2.1 hours; and Client #26, 2.0 hours) were run to criteria of two to ten-minute periods at 0 SW/M.

The data from Van Kirk (1972) are very impressive. She employed the DAF Program with criterion levels of five minutes at 0 SW/M. She consistently achieved elimination of stuttering (.3 SW/M) in the clinical setting with an average of 6.9 total therapy hours.

We view the DAF Program as one of the most powerful establishment programs available to us in operant stuttering therapy. Its effect is dramatic and quite consistent across clients. For best

TABLE VII

RESULTS OF PROGRAM 2, DELAYED AUDITORY FEEDBACK (DAF)

			Pre Means of Stuttered Words per Minute			Hours of Talking Time in Program	Post Means of Stuttered Words per Minute		
Clients	*Age*	*Sex*	*Reading*	*Monologue*	*Conversation*		*Reading*	*Monologue*	*Conversation*
1. RA	8	M	9.1	10.1	10.6	11.3	0	.1	.1
2. JA_2*	13	M		10.1	12.6	27.5		0	.1
3. DCo_2*	23	M	3.8		3.0	15.2	5.5		2.6
4. DH_2*	22	M	4.6	5.9	4.4	17.7	1.8	3.6	2.8
5. SJ	21	M	30.1	25.3		50.3	0	.2	
6. GLo	15	M	42.6			12.1	.5		
7. ML	15	M	6.4	6.8	8.8	32.6	0	0	0
8. GL	20	M	32.3		23.7	104.7	0		0
9. SM	14	M	6.3	16.1		12.4	.7	.9	
10. DM	14	M	37.5	27.3		13.3	4.1	1.2	
11. EM	31	M	15.0	13.0	12.0	177.2	0	0	0
12. SN	18	M	2.9	2.3	1.5	11.8	0	0	0
13. LO	22	M	9.3			3.9	0		
14. SP	25	F	13.0	11.0	11.6	97.7	.1	.9	.4
15. DPe	38	M	3.1	2.9	3.4	26.3	0	0	0
16. NW	33	M	10.3			8.4	.3		
17. BS	12	M	12.3	6.3	5.9	40.5	.5	.3	.5
18. RS	21	M	7.7	5.9	5.8	60.3	0	0	0
19. RW_2*	21	M	.5	1.5	1.8	29.0	.4	.2	.5
20. FF	45	M	2.8	1.4	1.2	2.5	0	0	0
21. WH	24	M	9.0	9.1	17.0	5.1	2.0	0	1.0
22. JS	43	M	26.0	14.0	10.0	7.5	.4	1.0	.3
23. DS	21	M	10.0	5.0	11.4	2.1	0	0	0
24. HN	35	M	4.8	2.0	3.4	13.3	0	0	0
25. JN	32	M	15.4	8.9	11.2	4.3	0	0	.1
26. PR	19	M	8.0	14.9	19.0	2.0	0	0	0
27. RL	18	M	15.9			5.2	0		
28. JB	17	M	8.2	10.9	14.8	4.7	0	.5	.3
Mean	22.9		12.8	9.6	9.2	28.6	.6	.4	.4
S.D.	9.4		11.1	6.9	6.2	39.4	1.3	.8	.8

* DCo, JA_2, DH_2 and RW_2 had been on Program 1, also.

results, however, it should be used in a systematic, programmed manner. Simply exposing a client to brief, random periods on the DAF machine may not produce positive changes.

Establishment Program 3: Punishment

An outline of the Punishment Program is shown in Figure 16. It is representative of the common simple punishment paradigm of following each stuttered word with an aversive (punishing) event. The program receives its name, of course, from the fact that the major characteristic of the procedure is the punishing event. If the event is functioning as a punisher, there will be a decrease in the frequency of stuttering.

In the Punishment Program, the client is instructed to read or monologue or converse and one or more of the aversive events are delivered contingent upon each stuttered word. The program is relatively easy to administer. The punishment process is continued until the stuttering behavior disappears. Cancellation of the stuttered word may also be used (Haroldson, Martin and Starr, 1968). The amount of punishment may also be varied. For example, if time-out is used, the period may be varied from ten seconds to one second. Branching would be used with these variables. The client's performance in this program is usually a relatively quick decrease in stuttering behavior within the first session which the client may achieve by slowing down, prolonging or doing whatever is necessary to speak fluently. Failure on a post-program Criterion Test would indicate a recycling through the program, probably at a lower amplitude of punishing events at reduced time periods. The minimal run time is unknown.

Step	*Stimulus*	*Response*	*Consequence*
1	Instructions to read.	Read.	Some aversive event. "Time-out," or "No," or replay tape with stuttering, or shock, or others.
2	Instructions to monologue.	Monologue.	Same.
3	Instructions to converse.	Converse.	Same.

Figure 16. Outline of Program 3, Punishment.

The goal of this program is to produce an attention to stuttering which the client will use to control the stuttering and learn to speak fluently. This internalized ability is a detection, pause and in some cases a cancelling process. Siegel (1970) refers to it as a *highlighting* process. Wingate (1959) also noted a decrease in stuttering rate as a function of simply counting or identifying stuttered words.

The finding that punishment reduced stuttering was first reported by Flanagan, Goldiamond and Azrin (1958) and followed by Martin and Siegel (1966a; 1966b). A number of different aversive events including response cost, coughing, noise, saying "tree" or "wrong," delayed auditory feedback, shock and counting stuttered words overtly may serve as punishers (Siegel, 1970; Cooper, Cady and Robbins, 1970; Murray, 1969; Quist and Martin, 1967; Toomey and Sidman, 1970; Williams, 1962; Halvorson, 1971; Gross and Holland, 1965; Daly and Frick, 1970; Webster and Dorman, 1970; Felty, 1959).

Time-out is an especially powerful, effective, and easily administered punishing event. It has been studied extensively (Martin, 1968; Siegel, 1970; Haroldson, Martin and Starr, 1968; 1971; Martin and Haroldson, 1969; 1971; Martin and Berndt, 1970; Egolf, Shames and Seltzer, 1971). The results have uniformly shown a reduction in the frequency of stuttering behavior.

Additional research on punishment and stuttering or normal disfluencies in normal speakers is summed up and analyzed by Martin (1968) and Siegel (1970). Their results indicate that punishment decreases normal disfluencies in normal speakers, also. This finding has raised many questions concerning the role of punishment in the acquisition and maintenance of stuttering. Much early literature as exemplified by Johnson et al. (1956) and Van Riper (1954) and recent research summaries such as Van Riper (1971) and Sheehan (1970) imply that punishment produces stuttering. Brutten and Shoemaker (1967) feel that punishment serves to elicit negative conditioned emotionality which in turn results in fluency failure. Biggs and Sheehan (1969) in a partial replication of the original Flanagan, Goldiamond and Azrin study interpreted their results to mean that distraction rather than punishment produced the decrease in stuttering.

Shames (1970) reminded his reader that much of stuttering therapy is already composed of punishing events such as asking the stutterer to repeat stuttered words (cancellation), to talk in unpleasant situations, etc. The controversy continues and is not yet resolved. There is an element of punishment in any program for stuttering, especially those which include an identification phase. Wingate (1959) observed a decrease in stuttering when attention was drawn to stuttering through a large counter placed in front of the subjects. There is usually a drop in stuttering rate when self-identification procedures are instituted in a program. It may further be speculated that the cancellation procedures advocated by Van Riper (1954; 1963) and programmed by Ryan (1964) serve to reduce stuttering frequency partly because of a punishment element. Many procedures such as watching oneself in the mirror, evaluating one's stuttering behavior, etc. may in reality act as punishing events. The author used instant replay television in a small study of people who stuttered. Fluent sentences were not replayed but only stuttered ones. A decrease in stuttering occurred. The whole concept of punishment and its role in stuttering etiology and more germanely its role in therapy, needs to be reanalyzed. The common result of punishment procedures is a marked decrease in the stuttering rate. Although some clients demonstrate a more gradual effect.

In Table VIII are shown the results for the Punishment Program with two clients. This program was quite effective. We have 17.0 hours of run time. Unlike others who used carefully controlled two-room administration of punishment we met with the two clients in a face-to-face situation and conversed with them or listened to their monologue. As a result, the clinicians tended to react normally during the time periods when the clients were not stuttering. The normal reaction often took the form of laughing and smiling. In short, we incidentally introduced some positive reinforcement for fluency at the same time as we were punishing stuttering.

For Client DH_3 the punishing event was a replay of the tape recorder after a stuttered word. Each time he stuttered, the tape recorder was rewound and he received an instant replay of his stuttered word. For Client DC, we used, "No," contingent on each

TABLE VIII

RESULTS OF PROGRAM 3, PUNISHMENT

			Pre Means of Stuttered Words per Minute			Hours of Talking Time in Program	Post Means of Stuttered Words per Minute		
Clients	Age	Sex	Reading	Monologue	Conversation		Reading	Monologue	Conversation
1. DC	15	M		12.1	13.9	6.1		.1	.7
2. DH_3*	20	M	3.0	5.1	4.0	10.3	.4	.4	.3
Mean	17.5		3.0	8.6	8.9	8.2	.4	.2	.5
S.D.	3.5		0	4.9	7.0	2.9	0	.2	.3

* DH_3 had been on Programs 1 and 2.

stuttered word. The two different punishers produced a significant reduction in stuttering.

Client BH who is reported in the next section under Establishment Program 4 also received a partial punishment program. We positively reinforced him for fluency (gave him a point) and punished him (removed a point) for each stuttered word. We included him in the next program section because the major characteristics of his treatment program were positive reinforcement and the control of response length and complexity.

These data and those generated by others previously cited appear to support the observation that punishment, defined as the administration of an aversive event contingent upon each stuttered word, is a very powerful way to reduce the frequency of stuttering behavior. The controversy over punishment tends to lie more in the theoretical, semantic and philosophical area rather than in the functional.

Establishment Program 4: Gradual Increase in Length and Complexity of Utterance

An outline of the Gradual Increase in Length and Complexity of Utterance Program or GILCU is shown in Figure 17. The complete program will be found elsewhere (Ryan and Van Kirk, 1971). This is a fifty-four step program which starts with reading a single word and works up to five minutes of fluent conversation. Hence, its name referring to the gradual increase in length and complexity of utterances. The words are changed constantly and the client is reinforced for each fluent novel response.

Should the client fail, be on one step without passing it for either three sessions or forty minutes, whichever comes first, the client is put on a branching program. The branch program for Establishment Program 4 is designed to use a model by the clinician of the client's response. If the client cannot generate fluent utterances, the clinician models them and gradually reduces the modeling through the various branch steps until the client can operate without the modeling at which time the client goes back on the program. If the client fails the post-program Criterion Test, the client is recycled through the program with a reduced

Step	*Stimulus*	*Response*
1	Instructions to read 1 word fluently.	1 word.
2	Instructions to read 2 words fluently.	2 words.
3-6	Instructions to read 3-6 words fluently.	3-6 words.
7-10	Instructions to read 1-4 sentences fluently.	1-4 sentences.
11-18	Instructions to read 30 seconds to 5 minutes fluently.	30 seconds to 5 minutes of reading.
19-54	Recycle in monologue and conversation.	Monologue or conversation.

Figure 17. Outline of Program 4, Gradual Increase in Length and Complexity of Utterance (GILCU).

criterion of performance during the program. The minimal run time is estimated at ninety minutes.

A second program (the Lea-Griffin Variations) is somewhat shorter. It focuses on speaking (echoing, monologue, naming, and conversation). It can be found elsewhere (Ryan, 1971). A third program (Van Kirk Variation) is a very comprehensive elaboration of the basic program which focuses on echoing, monologue, and conversation, and excludes reading. Her program varies the speech situations rather than the utterance length. It can also be found elsewhere (Ryan, 1971). Both of these two program variations have the one special advantage of holding the interest of very young children, usually preschoolers, for whom they were intended. However, this same kind of attention may be achieved by the use of powerful reinforcers. Therefore, the basic GILCU Program is recommended. The other two variations are mentioned merely to give full scope to the data. All three programs were used in the collection of the data.

The GILCU Program is concerned with the development of fluent speech through the careful control of the evoking stimuli. These procedures have concentrated on starting with simple verbal tasks such as uttering one word. It is helpful for the child who is not very verbal to increase talking. These programs are characterized by a very low rate of stuttering throughout the procedure. We recommend this program for preschoolers. Some form of this program has existed in many previous therapies for children (Van Riper, 1954; 1963; Brutten and Shoemaker, 1967). Instructions to speak more slowly or easily, relax, etc. often accompanied the procedures. Such procedures were called "desensitization" activities by Van Riper (1959; 1963).

Rickard and Mundy (1965) reported the use of such a program with a young child who was put through a program of gradually increased length of utterance: words, phrases, sentences, etc. This program was successful in establishing fluent speech. Haugen (1967a) reported an unsuccessful experience with an eight-year-old male using a similar format. Leach (1969) worked with a twelve-year-old male and was successful in gradually increasing both the amount of talking and fluency using money as a reinforcer. Shaw and Shrum (1972) essentially replicated Leach's work with three stutterers with comparable results.

Mowrer (1971b) using this program developed word lists and other cueing devices for both the client and the clinician. He used a number of different reinforcers ranging from social to money. Most of the eleven clients he reported on demonstrated great improvement in fluency in relatively short periods of therapy time. Van Kirk (1972) also reported successful experience with this program.

A variation on this theme is the work of Shames and Egolf (1970) in which the controlling stimuli are first identified and then manipulated by the clinician in a systematic way. In a sense, each child gets an individually designed, sophisticated program to evoke and reinforce fluent utterances.

The important feature that this program demonstrates is an immediate, sudden decrease, in stuttering behavior to almost 0 SW/M in the first sessions. There is a gradual slight increase in SW/M as the person completes the program and the responses become more complex.

In Table IX are shown the results for the GILCU Program. The nine clients ranged in age from seven to thirty-five. We have accumulated 207 hours of run time on this program. It has the very special advantages of a high degree of success and little or no attention to the act of stuttering. It is seldom necessary to dis-

TABLE IX

RESULTS OF PROGRAM 4, GRADUAL INCREASE IN LENGTH AND COMPLEXITY OF UTTERANCE (GILCU)

			Pre Means of Stuttered Words per Minute			*Hours of Talking Time*	*Post Means of Stuttered Words per Minute*		
Clients	*Age*	*Sex*	*Reading*	*Monologue*	*Conversation*	*in Program*	*Reading*	*Monologue*	*Conversation*
1. CE*	7	F		.6	5.1	20.9		.2	.1
2. KF	16	M	14.3	13.0	10.5	22.3	0	0	0
3. CG	34	M		20.0		10.5		1.5	
4. MHo*	7	M		12.1	14.6	60.1		0	0
5. MLi*	8	M	4.2	3.2	2.4	9.7	0	0	0
6. CM	35	M	14.2	10.4	12.7	38.6	0	1.2	.5
7. JG	8	M			9.6	6.6			.5
8. BH	9	M	4.0	9.5	15.0	15.4	0	0	0
9. RM	8	M		10.3	11.0	25.3		0	0
Mean	14.7		9.2	9.9	10.1	23.2	0	.4	.1
S.D.	11.6		5.1	6.0	4.4	16.9	0	.6	.2

* CE, MHo and MLi were run on variations of the GILCU Program.

cuss stuttering behavior in this program. This is a special advantage for young children who are not yet aware of their stuttering. The GILCU Program has been demonstrated to be an effective program.

COMPARISON OF THE FOUR ESTABLISHMENT PROGRAMS

The data on all four Establishment Programs are summarized in Table X. Because the time periods and criterion levels varied so greatly, these figures give only some general indications of the relative merits of the programs. We certainly have little data (N 2) for the Punishment Program.

All of the programs produced a significant change in the frequency of stuttering in reading, monologue and conversation. The two longest running programs are the Delayed Auditory Feedback (a mean of 28.6 hours) and the Gradual Increase in Length and Complexity of Utterance (a mean of 23.2 hours). Examination of the performance of individual clients on recent, revised versions of these programs indicate that both of these programs can run quite quickly, less than ten hours of therapy time (Van Kirk, 1972; Ryan and Van Kirk, 1971).

Until definitive research has indicated which of the programs is the most effective in terms of time, fluency, transfer and maintenance, the clinician has the option of selecting those programs which best can be accomplished in his or her individual setting with the equipment and skills available to him or her.

There is another option. It is possible to construct a program that has all the components of all the programs. In Table XI all four programs are compared along the dimensions of stimuli, responses, criterion, consequences, end goal behavior and time. Note that all programs have an aversive consequence for stuttering. A fifth program which is a composite of the four is also described. It should teach everything in a very rapid manner with very little error. Until further research has indicated the relative merits of the individual programs, the omnibus program will have to wait.

Our goal is the development of a program which will consistently produce fluency in the greatest number of people who stutter in the shortest period of time. There are undoubtedly an

TABLE X

SUMMARY OF RESULTS OF ALL FOUR ESTABLISHMENT PROGRAMS

No. *Programs*	*Number of Clients*	*Age Mean*	*Pre Means of Stuttered Words per Minute*			*Post Means of Stuttered Words per Minute*			*Hours of Talking Time in Program Mean*
			Reading	*Monologue*	*Conversation*	*Reading*	*Monologue*	*Conversation*	
1. Programmed traditional	19	19.3	11.2	8.9	5.8	4.8	1.1	3.1	13.3
2. Delayed auditory feedback	28	22.9	12.8	9.6	9.2	.6	.4	.4	28.6
3. Punishment	2	17.5	3.0	8.6	8.9	.4	.2	.5	8.2
4. Gradual increase in length and complexity of utterance	9	14.7	9.2	9.9	10.1	0	.4	.1	23.2

TABLE XI

COMPARISON OF THE FOUR ESTABLISHMENT PROGRAMS ON SEVERAL VARIABLES AND A COMPOSITE PROGRAM

No.	Programs and Stimuli	Responses	Criterion	Consequences: Fluency	Consequences: Stuttering	End Goal Behaviors	Minimal Run Time (Minutes)
1.	Programmed traditional Instructions Modeling	Identification Cancellation Pullout Prolongation Fluency	Per cent correct Time at specified stuttering or fluency rate	"Good" and/or token	Instruction Identification	Can count SW Cancel Pullout Prolong Fluency	114
2.	Delayed auditory feedback Instructions DAF machine Modeling	Identification Stop and pause Fluency	Per cent correct Time at specified stuttering or fluency rate	"Good" and/or token	"Stop" Identification	Can count SW Stop and pause Fluency	111
3.	Punishment Instructions	Stop and pause Cancel Identification	Per cent correct Time at specified stuttering or fluency rate		T.O. (time out) "No"	Can count SW Cancel Stop and pause Fluency	Unknown
4.	Gradual increase in length and complexity of utterance Instructions	Stop and pause Fluency	Per cent correct Number of words, sentences Time fluent	"Good" and/or token	"Stop"	Can count SW Stop and pause Fluency	90 (Estimated)
5.	Composite Instructions DAF machine Modeling	Identification Stop and pause Cancel Prolongation Fluency	Per cent correct Time at specified fluency rate Number of words, sentences Time fluent	"Good" and/or token	T.O. (time out) "Stop" Identification	Can count SW Stop and pause Cancel Prolong Fluency	111

infinite number of programs possible, but the question is, are there any programs truly different from or better than any of the four already described?

SUMMARY

In this Chapter four Establishment Programs: Program 1, Programmed Traditional; Program 2, Delayed Auditory Feedback; Program 3, Punishment; and Program 4, Gradual Increase in Length and Complexity of Utterance were described. Data were presented to demonstrate the effects of each of these programs. They all resulted in the decrease in frequency of stuttering behavior. A comparison was made of all four programs. It is not yet clear which program is best. An omnibus program was suggested.

CHAPTER VI

PROGRAMS: TRANSFER AND MAINTENANCE

THIS CHAPTER IS DEVOTED to the discussion of programs for the transfer and maintenance of fluent speech after it has once been established in the clinic room setting. The programs, with modifications, apply to both children and adults. Although no hard and fast rules hold we commonly define children as those clients under thirteen and define adults as those thirteen or older. Factors such as severity, speaking needs and home cooperation must also be taken into consideration when carrying out transfer programs for children and adults.

TRANSFER

Transfer—The goal in this phase is fluent speech in a wide variety of settings with many different people.

Bandura (1969) suggests that there are three areas of interest for transfer of training: 1) a special transfer of training procedure, 2) self-regulatory activities taught to the client and 3) changing the environmental reaction to present behavior.

Commonly, in traditional therapy for people who stutter it has been expected that they would transfer or carryover their new fluency to all the settings they need. It was assumed that the person had learned some self-regulatory skills. In the treatment of children, clinicians attempted to produce environmental change through helping their parents react differently. Reports by Prins (1970), Gregory (1969) and Van Riper (1958) and observation by any clinician who has worked with stutterers over long time periods have shown that these somewhat casual transfer and maintenance procedures have not been successful. We apparently need to program the use of fluent speech in settings other than the clinic. Indeed, there may be a danger in over-training in the clinic setting in that such over-training might actually interfere with transfer (Mowrer, 1971c).

In our early operant work with people who stuttered we, too, assumed that once the clients had learned fluent speech in the clinic they would spontaneously transfer. Our finding was that this was seldom true even though the people had demonstrated very fluent speech (0 SW/M) over long time periods (an hour a day, five days a week, for over one hundred hours of training). Extensive fluency experiences in the clinic setting did not insure fluency in the world. There were exceptions to this observation. Most children and some adults did spontaneously transfer their new fluent speech. Most adults and some children did not.

In developing a Transfer Program a first order decision concerned whether to choose reciprocal inhibition procedures which emphasized the visualization of various speaking situations, (Wolpe, 1958; 1969; Gray and England, 1969; 1972; Gray, 1969; Lanyon, 1969; Brutten and Shoemaker, 1967) or an actual participation *in vivo* of the person in a wide variety of speaking situations. Our choice was the latter. Although reciprocal inhibition done in the clinic setting may be a more economical use of the clinician's time, it is still necessary to measure the speech in the actual setting to determine whether or not the visualization procedure has been effective.

The Transfer Program to be described is composed of *in situ* procedures in which the person who stutters actually performs in a wide variety of settings. Transfer was separated from maintenance. Transfer refers to the acquisition of the fluent speech response in a wide variety of settings whereas maintenance refers to the continued use of fluent speech over time. These seemed to be two separate events because several clients who demonstrated excellent fluency in both establishment and transfer phases of therapy were unable to maintain it.

We have developed a Transfer Program for two reasons: 1) to measure the effects of the Establishment Programs and 2) to help the client transfer fluent speech. For the Transfer Program we will describe, it is not possible to separate the individual influences of the two procedures. The process of monitoring the effects of the program and the therapeutic effects of the monitoring process are intermixed. When it is possible through new electronic devices or other covert procedures (Andrews and Ingham, 1971) to monitor the client's speech without the client knowing it, we may find out the differential effects. At the moment, therapeutically and functionally, it is helpful to engage in the Transfer Program. It is also possible that some time in the future when we have more data or more sophisticated establishment procedures we shall not need such an extensive Transfer Program. In the future it may not be necessary for all clients to go through Transfer Programs.

In the development of the Transfer Program we have tried to consider the basic speaking experiences and settings a client might engage in and to include all the factors suggested by Bandura (1969). We developed a Transfer Program which attempts to teach the client to become self-regulatory in fluency skills. The Transfer Program also provides for a change of the environmental reaction to the client's fluency through the use of special instruction to selected audiences such as peers, parents and teachers.

Regardless of the type of Establishment Program the client has been on, the client will have some skill in conversational fluency. The client may or may not have already indicated signs of transfer by the time the Establishment Program has been completed. If so, the client will go very quickly and easily through the Transfer Program. In this event, the Transfer Program will have value mainly as a measurement procedure. If the client has not shown signs of transfer, then the Transfer Program becomes critical to provide transfer.

Home Practice

A preliminary step in transfer is home practice. It is not included in the Transfer Program proper because we find it a hard variable to control and the Transfer Program will run without it. Home practice consists of the client practicing reading and/or monologue and/or conversation each day throughout the Establishment Program. The client gradually fades out practice at home during the transfer period and practices only when necessary during the maintenance period. Home practice is viewed as replicating the clinic procedure at home with the client or the parent or spouse as the observer. It is the client's first opportunity to take what was learned in the clinic setting and apply it elsewhere. It is important that this practice is monitored. We insist that clients tape record their home practice or at least keep a record of their practice time and the number of stuttered words they counted (see Home Practice Sheet in Figure 18). The client needs the skill to count stuttered words. This is taught directly in only three programs: Programs 1—Programmed Traditional; 2—Delayed Auditory Feedback; and 3—Punishment. After completion of Program 4, Gradual Increase in Length and Complexity of Utterance, the client may or may not be able to count stuttered words. The client may engage in home practice without counting stuttered words or may be taught to count them at the time of implementation of the home practice activities. For younger clients or other clients who cannot learn to count stuttered words, we teach the parent or spouse to count stuttered words.

The clients, generally only older children and adults, are instructed to parallel the clinic program at home. If they are working on reading in the Establishment Program at the clinic or school, they are to practice reading for five minutes daily at home at the outset of therapy. When they get to monologue at the clinic, they now can reduce their reading practice to two minutes and add five minutes of monologue practice. When they reach conversation they can reduce their reading and monologue to two minutes each and add five minutes of conversation with some member of their family or a friend.

We recommend home practice as being very helpful in both the establishment and transfer of fluent speech. Others such as Peins, Lee and McGough (1970) have presented data on the helpful effects of home tape recorder practice. However, we are aware that it may be difficult for the clinician to monitor the home practice and/or to motivate the client to carry it out. An initial verbal contract with the client that purchase or the loan of a tape recorder (inexpensive cassettes are adequate) and that consistent home practice are vital to the therapy program has often been enough to encourage this. The client is asked to bring in the home tape recordings each session and we do monitor each

HOME PRACTICE RECORD Name______________________

Date	Session Number	Activity	Time	Total Stuttered Words	SW/M	Date	Session Number	Activity	Time	Total Stuttered Words	SW/M

Figure 18. Home Practice Record (Reprinted with permission from Behavioral Sciences Institute, Monterey, California, copyright, 1971.

one and report our observations to the client. This provides reinforcement to the client for having done them and information for us about their accuracy.

The fluency programs will work without home practice. The Transfer Program is designed to help those clients who are unable to help themselves through home practice. If the home practice period cannot be monitored, it is better to bypass this activity and continue with the Transfer Program which eventually involves the home setting.

Transfer Program

In Figure 19 is shown an outline of the Transfer Program (Ryan, 1970). We have used this Transfer Program or parts of it for several years now and have data on fifteen clients. It is difficult to give an accurate statement about the length of Transfer Programs because they have varied with individuals. However, our latest version (Ryan and Van Kirk, 1971) requires between ten to fifteen hours of therapy time.

Some clients, especially children, will have begun to transfer their new fluent speech *spontaneously,* especially if they have been on home practice periods. The clinician should attempt to measure this spontaneous transfer by interviewing the client and the people in the environment and observing the client in a number of different settings. Even if there are signs of transfer, it is usually a good idea to go through the entire Transfer Program.

Most of the transfer steps are in the conversation mode with some monologue in the large group settings. The clinician should give the same instructions as in the conversation part of the Establishment Program, i.e. "Speak Fluently," etc. A criterion level should be set for each step commonly five to ten consecutive minutes of fluent speech (0 SW/M). Only social reinforcement is given during the Transfer Program.

Series A. Physical Setting

In this series the clinician goes around to various places with the client engaging him in conversation. The steps are small to prevent relapse and to permit success.

Step	*Stimulus*	*Response*
Series A: Physical settings		
1	Clinician. Clinic room with door open.	Conversation.
2	Clinician. Immediately outside the clinic room.	Conversation.
3	Clinician. Down the hall from the clinic room.	Conversation.
4	Clinician. Outside the building of the clinic room.	Conversation.
5	Clinician. Walking around the building of the clinic room.	Conversation.
6	Clinician. In different rooms in other buildings.	Conversation.
Series B: Audience size		
1	One additional person in clinic room, does not interact.	Conversation.
2	One additional person in clinic room, does interact.	Conversation.
3	Two additional people in clinic room, do not interact.	Conversation.
4	Two additional people in clinic room, do interact.	Conversation.
5-8	Continue, up to five people.	Conversation.
9	Speech to group of five.	Speech.
10	Speech to group of ten.	Speech.
11	Speech to group of fifteen.	Speech.
Series C: Strangers and physical setting		
1	Various strangers in different physical settings with clinician close at hand.	Conversation.
2	Various strangers in different physical settings with clinician at a distance.	Conversation.
3	Various strangers in different settings without the clinician.	Conversation and reports to clinician.
Series D: Telephone		
1	Clinician.	Pretend phone is present.
2	Fake telephone with clinician.	Call, answer and converse.

Step	*Stimulus*	*Response*
3	Real telephone with clinician.	Call, answer and converse.
4	Real telephone with friends and/or relatives.	Call, answer and converse.
5	Real telephone with strangers.	Call, answer and converse.
Series E: Natural environment		
1	School, teacher and peers with and without clinician.	Conversation.
2	Home, parent and siblings with and without clinician.	Conversation.
3	Work, boss and fellow employees with and without clinician.	Conversation.

Figure 19. Outline of Transfer Program.

Series B. Audience Size

The purpose of this series is to gradually and systematically increase the number of listeners and conversational partners. This audience could be strangers, friends, relatives, spouses, teachers, classmates, or even other persons who stuttered provided that they, too, were at the same level of fluency. These may be the same people all the way through or new people may be introduced in each situation. These people may be trained to reinforce fluency and/or to count stuttered words. Parents and spouses may be brought into this series.

Series C. Strangers and Physical Settings

The client and clinician should first make a list of the speaking situations with strangers which the client commonly avoids or in which he finds himself. This list will vary with the age of the client and the daily communication activities. Ideally, these should be real situations arranged in a sequence of easy to hard according to the client's and the clinician's judgment about them. Commonly, these situations should be with a number of different people, rather than for longer periods with just a few. If the client is unable to construct such a list, the clinician should be ready to make up one which covers a number of different speaking situations appropriate to the age and/or interests of the client. In order to carry out steps two and three of this series the client must be able to monitor or count stuttered words. This series is probably not as critical with younger children as it is with older children and adults.

Series D. Telephone

This series is of value to older children and adults who use the telephone or would use it, if they were fluent. For some adults who show extreme fear of the telephone a number of substeps such as simply saying, "Hi" or "Hello" or "Goodbye," may be necessary. It is helpful to have a list of telephone numbers prepared ahead of time to avoid wasting time looking through a telephone book. Ideally, these should be real telephone situations concerning actual interests of the client. However, often they have to be contrived to collect enough of them. Clients occasionally voice concern about bothering merchants with fake telephone calls. However, the telephone calls themselves and the telephone series itself are not excessively long.

Series E. Natural Environments

Some of the preceding steps in the Transfer Program may have already touched the natural environment by going to familiar places and bringing in friends and relatives. The clinician acts more as an observer than as a conversational partner in these settings. The teacher or parent or spouse may be trained to reinforce the client for fluent speech in these settings. The work environment will, of course, be limited to those clients who are employed. It is occasionally offensive to a client to have the clinician in the work or school environment. In such instances the client must be trained to do the step alone and count stuttered words.

The client may also make tape recordings in these settings which can be shared with the clinician at a later time. The clinician may also interview people in the client's school or home or work environment to determine the success of the client in those settings.

Branching

Failure on the Transfer Program is three sessions or forty minutes on one step. The branching sequence in the Transfer Programs refers to having the clinician do anything that would be helpful to the client. Often, it is a few more substeps in the series.

Other Transfer Procedures

There are many other transfer procedures possible. Brutten and Shoemaker (1967) among others, suggest extensive, individualized hierarchies of visualized speaking experiences which may include seventy to one hundred different steps. Our experience, as borne out by the data in the next few pages, indicates that the steps in the present Transfer Program are usually enough for most clients. It is possible that the *in situ* experience is more powerful than the visualized experience.

Monitoring people during transfer procedures or activities is greatly enhanced by portable, wireless FM microphones. Our experience with such equipment has been that observations have been made much easier by the use of this equipment. The FM microphone transmits to a tape recorder-receiver which the clinician can monitor and/or tape record for later monitoring. Hence, the clinician may stand next to the client in transfer situations and tape record the experience covertly or stand some one hundred feet away and monitor and/or tape record.

With one client, a dentist, the FM microphone was placed on him while he went about his dentistry and talking. He changed the tape on the tape recorder himself to permit an hour and a half of tape recording. The microphone did not interfere with his activities, encouraged him to remember to speak fluently and gave us data on transfer of fluency.

Transfer Data

We have carried out some form of Transfer Program with twenty-two of our fifty-eight cases. With those clients who went through extensive, complete Transfer Programs (N 15), we carefully measured their stuttering rate. For those whom we put through only a partial program, our only measure was casual observation. Finally, there were twenty-eight clients whom we did not put through a Transfer Program. It also was not possible to measure their speech in environments other than the clinic room.

In our early work with people who stuttered we focused more on Establishment Programs. The Transfer Programs were initiated later, hence, it was not possible to put all our clients through Transfer Programs as a number of them had moved or left the program for other reasons.

In Table XII are shown the results of the fifteen clients whose speech in transfer activities was measured.

The actual transfer procedures varied greatly from client to client. For clients JA and RA, transfer reflected talking in their classroom. For client SJ, transfer consisted of ten-minute daily practice sessions with his wife. For client BH we focused on his family (Ryan, 1971). We experimented with many different forms of transfer. The Transfer Program shown earlier in Figure 19 represents a compilation of the best parts of all of the previous experimental models. The most recent version of the Transfer Program, with performance data, will be found in Ryan and Van Kirk (1971).

It can be seen in Table XII that the clients transferred their low rate of stuttering from the Establishment Programs to the

TABLE XII

RESULTS OF TRANSFER PROGRAM

Client	*Age*	*Sex*	*Talking Time in Minutes*	*Means of Stuttered Words per Minute During Transfer*
1. RA	9	M	135	.3
2. JA	14	M	1300	.6
3. DC	15	M	353	.2
4. DHo	22	M	420	.7
5. BH	9	M	113	.01
6. MHo	7	M	410	.7
7. SJ	21	M	2160	.05
8. ML	15	M	210	.4
9. SS	14	M	2760	.8
10. DS	21	M	56	.2
11. HN	35	M	106	.4
12. JN	32	M	227	.2
13. JB	17	M	49	.3
14. JS	43	M	200	1.0
15. WH	21	M	43	1.4
Mean	19.9		569.5	.5
S.D.	10.2		835.1	.4

speaking situations in the Transfer Program. This demonstrates the effects of the Establishment Programs.

Van Kirk (1972), using similar transfer procedures, reported that for eighteen clients a mean of .09 SW/M with a S.D. of .08 was achieved. This was accomplished with a mean of 6.9 therapy hours and a S.D. of 5.1 hours in transfer activity.

MAINTENANCE

Maintenance—The goal in this phase is fluent speech in a wide variety of settings, with many different people over a long period of time (several years).

Maintenance, as did Transfer, has two functions: 1) to measure the client's continued fluency and 2) to aid in helping the client maintain fluency. We have used several different strategies for maintenance. The basic one has been to gradually fade out the number of therapy activities until such time that the client can direct the therapy or does not need it.

Three kinds of activities have been involved in our maintenance procedure: 1) self-control through counting stuttered words each day in the environment, 2) intermittent home practice (discussed as a pretransfer activity) and 3) clinic contact for measurement and reinstruction.

Home Practice

If the client had been doing home practice, this was gradually faded out during the Transfer Program and was continued at low frequency during Maintenance. This was done to encourage a client to improve fluency in the world, to help the client see the progress being made and to provide data on fluency. During Maintenance, clients used home practice only if they had a *bad day* and wanted to regain their fluency skills. Parents used it occasionally when their children were going through a *bad spell*. Home practice was used for additional fluency practice, faded out and finally, evoked only when failure was observed.

Counting Stuttered Words

We have used the procedure of asking a client to count each

stuttered word each day. Some clients wore wrist counters and dutifully counted each stuttered word each day. These data were recorded on a chart. This was considered part of the self-monitoring or self-control system. It was gradually faded out.

Clinic Contact

Clinic contact was also gradually faded out. The clinic contact generally was composed of collecting a sample of the client's speech and asking about the client's speaking experience in the world. Occasionally, additional training sessions were scheduled based on the client's performance.

We evolved a rather elaborate schedule for producing a systematic fade of each of the three events; home practice, clinic contact and daily count. This schedule is shown in Figure 20. This very elaborate schedule is of value in a research oriented ac-

Week	*Home-Practice (Number per Week)*	*Clinic (Number per Week)*	*Count (Number per Week)*
1	7	3	7
2	6	2	6
3	5	1	6
4	4	1	4
5	3	1	3
6	2	1	2
7	1	0	1
8	1	1	1
9	1	0	1
10	1	1	1
11	0	0	0
12	1	0	1
13	0	1	0
14	1	0	1
15	1	0	0
16	0	0	0
17	0	1	1
18	0	0	0
19	0	0	0
20	0	0	0
21	1	1	1
25	1	1	1
29	1	1	1
37	1	1	1
59	1	1	1
Total	40	18	40

Figure 20. Maintenance Program schedule for 59 weeks (14 months).

tivity and should probably be explored. Our basic finding was that it was not particularly helpful and quite complicated to maintain.

Maintenance Program

Therefore, we developed a more simplified version of the Maintenance Program (Ryan and Van Kirk, 1971) shown in outline form in Figure 21. This program is written in the same format as the Establishment and Transfer Programs. It provides for clinic rechecks which are gradually faded out over a two-year period. The collection of a sample of reading, monologue and conversation during each session provides for a measurement of the client's progress. A rate above .5 SW/M indicates the need for additional training. The client may also be queried as to fluency in other environments and additional training in reported difficult situations such as talking on the telephone and giving public speeches may be instituted. This is a form of branching. This much simpler procedure has been equally effective and much easier to administer. It meets the requirements of gradual fading, providing for measurement of post-program speech fluency and providing clinic contact to determine if the client still needs additional help or retraining.

Step	*Stimulus*	*Response*
Series A:		
1-4	Four weekly meetings.	Read, monologue, converse and report.
5	One month later.	Read, monologue, converse and report.
6	Three months later.	Read, monologue, converse and report.
7	Six months later.	Read, monologue, converse and report.
8	Twelve months later.	Read, monologue, converse and report.

Figure 21. Outline of Maintenance Program.

Maintenance Data

It has been possible to carry out long term Maintenance Programs with only nine clients (JA, JB, SS, HN, FF, JS, DS, CE, and BH). Each of these maintenance procedures was somewhat different although basically they were composed of gradually decreasing practice periods and contact with the clinic during which time the procedures were reviewed. They varied in overall length from three to forty months.

The Maintenance Program for the clients included personal contact, telephone calls, postcards, and tape recordings made by the client and sent to the clinician for analysis. The critical feature is that the clinician must stay in touch with the client. For client SS, it was found during maintenance activities that he needed further training. The parents of BH needed additional reinforcement to keep up their practice periods. The maintenance phase of therapy is very important.

It was possible to follow-up twenty-four clients. The results of this follow-up are shown in Table XIII. Both children and adults were included in this sample. Most of the clients had been on Establishment Program No. 2, Delayed Auditory Feedback. The average age of the clients was twenty years. They demonstrated a pre-program stuttering rate of a mean of 9.9 SW/M and a post-program stuttering rate of a mean of .3 SW/M. The follow-up check which was done live on sixteen clients and from tape recordings on eight clients (RS, BS, SS, ML, JN, HN, BH and EM) demonstrated a stuttering rate of a mean of 1.7 SW/M. Seven clients (JA, SP, RS, BS, DPe, EM and ML) had received some type of therapy during the intervening period. This therapy varied in both amount and focus and was not operant in any formal sense.

We had put sixteen of the clients through transfer activities. Nine of them had been on a Maintenance Program. All of the clients demonstrated a lower stuttering rate during the follow-up check than their pre-program rate, however, three of them (JA, SP, and SJ) demonstrated relatively high rates during the recheck indicating relapse. All three of them had been through some kind of Transfer Program, but only one (JA) had been on a Maintenance Program. Using a criterion of 1 SW/M it can be seen that fourteen of the clients maintained. Half of these were children. Six clients demonstrated fluency at 0 SW/M.

In order to further analyze the effects of Transfer and Maintenance Programs on long term fluency an additional analysis of the older clients (aged fourteen to forty-five) was made. It was

TABLE XIII

RESULTS OF FOLLOW-UP

Client	Age	Sex	Pre Means of Stuttered Words per Minute	Post Means of Stuttered Words per Minute	Number of Months Since End of Program	Means of Stuttered Words per Minute at Follow-up	Had Transfer Program	Had Maintenance Program
1. JA	14	M	11.3	.1	8	7.8	Yes	Yes
2. SP	25	F	11.8	.4	8	9.3	Yes	No
3. CE	7	F	2.8	0	8	0	No	Yes
4. RS	21	M	6.4	0	20	1.3	No	No
5. JG	8	M	9.6	.5	8	.3	No	No
6. BS	12	M	8.1	.4	20	0	Yes	No
7. SJ	21	M	27.7	.2	8	8.7	Yes	No
8. DPe	28	M	3.1	0	8	.4	No	No
9. MHo	7	M	13.3	0	8	.5	No	No
10. MLi	8	M	3.3	0	8	.2	No	No
11. SS	14	M	14.0	.5	40	.2	Yes	Yes
12. ML	15	M	7.3	0	4	.3	Yes	No
13. JN	32	M	11.8	0	1	.7	Yes	No
14. HN	35	M	3.4	0	3	.1	Yes	Yes
15. FF	45	M	1.8	0	23	0	Yes	Yes
16. JS	43	M	16.6	.8	12	2.4	Yes	Yes
17. DS	21	M	8.8	0	10	0	Yes	Yes
18. MH	20	M	9.1	1.5	24	0	Yes	No
19. DC	15	M	13.0	.7	3	1.3	Yes	No
20. WH	24	M	11.8	1.0	1	3.0	Yes	No
21. RA	8	M	9.9	.1	3	1.1	No	No
22. BH	9	M	9.5	0	21	0	Yes	Yes
23. EM	31	M	13.3	0	20	2.0	No	No
24. JB	17	M	11.3	.3	6	1.3	Yes	Yes
Mean	20.0		9.9	.3	11.5	1.7		
S.D.	11.1		5.5	.4	9.4	2.8		
Total "Yes"							16	9
Total "No"							8	15

decided to exclude younger clients in this analysis because our observation had been that most of the children transferred *spontaneously* without an extensive Transfer Program.

Transfer Programs were subjectively divided into the categories of partial and complete. Partial transfer meant that some transfer activities had been conducted whereas complete transfer meant that the entire Transfer Program shown in Figure 19 had been carried out. A criterion of 1 SW/M was used to determine whether or not the clients had maintained their speech fluency. The results of this analysis are shown in Table XIV.

In the no transfer and maintenance group (N 3) only one of the clients had maintained. The client, DPe, had entered the program with a relatively low rate of 3.1 SW/M and still demonstrated some stuttering, .4 SW/M, during the follow-up check.

In the partial transfer and no maintenance group (N 5) only one of the clients had maintained. Interestingly enough that client, MH, had initially demonstrated quite severe stuttering (9.1 SW/M) with much struggle behavior. However, the transfer activities, because of our lack of knowledge at that time, were spread over a twelve-month period and could be viewed as a combination of transfer and maintenance.

In the partial transfer and maintenance group (N 4) only one of the clients had maintained. The client, FF, had entered the program with a fairly low rate of stuttering (1.8 SW/M) composed mostly of struggle behavior. He was very diligent about home practice and spent many hours reading and speaking on his tape recorder. All of the three clients who did not maintain had difficulty during the partial transfer activities. We questioned at the time if they were really fluent enough for transfer procedures, but put them through anyway. The results suggest that they should have spent more time in the Establishment Program.

In the complete transfer and no maintenance group (N 2) both of the clients had maintained their fluency at the follow-up three months later which was a rather short period.

In the complete transfer and maintenance group (N 3) all three of the clients maintained their fluency on the average of seventeen months, however, the months of maintenance ranged from three to forty.

TABLE XIV

RESULTS OF FOLLOW-UP FOR FIVE GROUPS

Group	Clients	Means of Stuttered Words per Minute Pre	Post	Follow-up	Means of Months of Follow-up	Number of Clients Maintained at Less Than 1 SW/M	Total
1. No transfer, no maintenance	EM, RS, DPe	7.7	0	5.1	8	1	3
2. Partial transfer, no maintenance	SP, ST, MH, DC, WH	14.7	.7	4.4	9	1	5
3. Partial transfer, maintenance	JS, FF, JB, JA	9.9	.2	3.5	10	1	4
4. Complete transfer, no maintenance	ML, JN	9.2	0	.5	3	2	2
5. Complete transfer, maintenance	DS, SS, HN	8.4	.2	.2	17	3	3

The conclusion that may be drawn from these limited data is that Transfer and Maintenance Programs are necessary to transfer and maintain fluency established in the clinic setting. In further support of this hypothesis, Van Kirk (1972) using similar transfer and maintenance procedures, reported that eighteen of her clients had maintained at a mean of .08 SW/M from two to twenty months. Andrews and Ingham (1971) report maintenance of fluency in their subjects. It is difficult to compare these data with other reports of follow-up (Gregory, 1969; Prins, 1969; Van Riper, 1958) because the procedures were different. Follow-up data undoubtedly are the single most important measure to determine the effectiveness of any system of therapy. Unfortunately, they are lacking in the literature both in quantity and precision.

There are some speculations which can be made about Transfer and Maintenance Programs. They, undoubtedly, are much too complex and too long. We probably do not need all of these procedures for all the clients with whom we are working. For example, preschool children may need only home procedures. We need to develop tests to place individuals in only those parts of the Transfer Program they need.

The most important part of the maintenance of a behavior may be the schedule of reinforcement (Skinner, 1953). How do we build Establishment and/or Transfer and/or Maintenance Programs which include that factor? Gradually fading out the contact is one form of gradually reducing the reinforcement schedule, but it may not be the most powerful. Built-in intermittent reinforcement during the Establishment and Transfer Programs may be the answer.

At this state of our knowledge, our data seem to suggest that we need Transfer and Maintenance Programs if for no other reason than to provide follow-up data on the effects of our Establishment Programs. The second reason we find more clinically tenable. Transfer and Maintenance Programs do indeed seem to provide for the transfer and maintenance of fluent speech.

SUMMARY

Transfer and Maintenance Programs were discussed and examples presented. Data to support their effectiveness were presented.

Transfer and maintenance activities are necessary for the measurement of the effectiveness of training and the transfer and maintenance of fluency.

CHAPTER VII

CLIENT PERFORMANCE IN PROGRAMS

IN THIS CHAPTER will be shown client performance in the four Establishment Programs and the Transfer and Maintenance Programs, client performance in unusual programs and an analysis of clients and programs which failed.

CLIENT PERFORMANCE IN THE FOUR ESTABLISHMENT PROGRAMS

The clients chosen for examples in each of the various programs were selected on the basis that they were successful and they went through establishment, transfer and maintenance phases. Audio tape recordings of the performance of these clients are on file with the author.

Program 1, Programmed Traditional, Stan (SS)

Stan was fourteen years old when he came to us from his home town some 150 miles away. He was the first client with whom we were to go through an entire Establishment, Transfer and Maintenance Program. His history has been shared earlier (Ryan, 1970; Ryan, 1968a).

The Establishment and most of the Transfer Program took place in a university clinic during an eight-week summer session in 1967. Base Rate (Criterion Test) data collected during the first two days revealed a rate of 4.0 SW/M in reading and 24.0 SW/M in speaking. His stuttering consisted of part-word repetition, whole word repetition and exhalation of air preceding words (struggle). The Base Rate and program data are shown on a linear chart in Figure 22.

Stan entered the Establishment Program the following day. He read or spoke for three hours a day, four days a week. Three different clinicians worked with him daily. All sessions were audio tape recorded. The three clinicians reached 90 per cent agreement among themselves on the counting of stuttered words.

The program to establish fluent reading, speaking, and conversation was essentially Program 1, Programmed Traditional. At the end of eight days in this program Stan was reading and engaging in monologue at less than 1 SW/M. A conversation period was added. Throughout the rest of the program Stan read, engaged in monologue and conversed daily.

The Transfer Program began in session 11. This program contained a gradual increase in audience size from two through fifty-six, a gradual increase in the complexity of the conversational setting including talking on the telephone, talking with strangers, talking in a wide variety of physical settings and group discussion. It was a prototype of our present Transfer Program. He also talked with his mother in the clinic. Throughout the Transfer Program he maintained a rate of less than 1 SW/M. At the end of twenty-five sessions (seventy-five therapy hours) Stan was speaking very fluently in a wide variety of situations as observed by himself, the clinicians and his parents.

The Maintenance Program began two weeks after the conclusion of the summer program. It took place in Stan's hometown, some 150 miles away from the clinic. It consisted of three activities: 1) weekly speech therapy sessions during which his local speech clinician continued to monitor his reading and speaking, 2) weekly home tape recording sessions during which Stan read, engaged in monologue and conversed in the presence of one or both of his parents, and 3) periodic one-session visits to the university clinic where his reading and speaking were measured and additional instructions were given. Program modifications were made at these university clinic rechecks. The home tape recordings were mailed in weekly by Stan to the clinic for analysis. A type-written analysis of the tape recording was returned to Stan. These tapes revealed significant increases in stuttering rate on three occasions. The home program was modified each time.

Home Program Modification I was the addition of client iden-

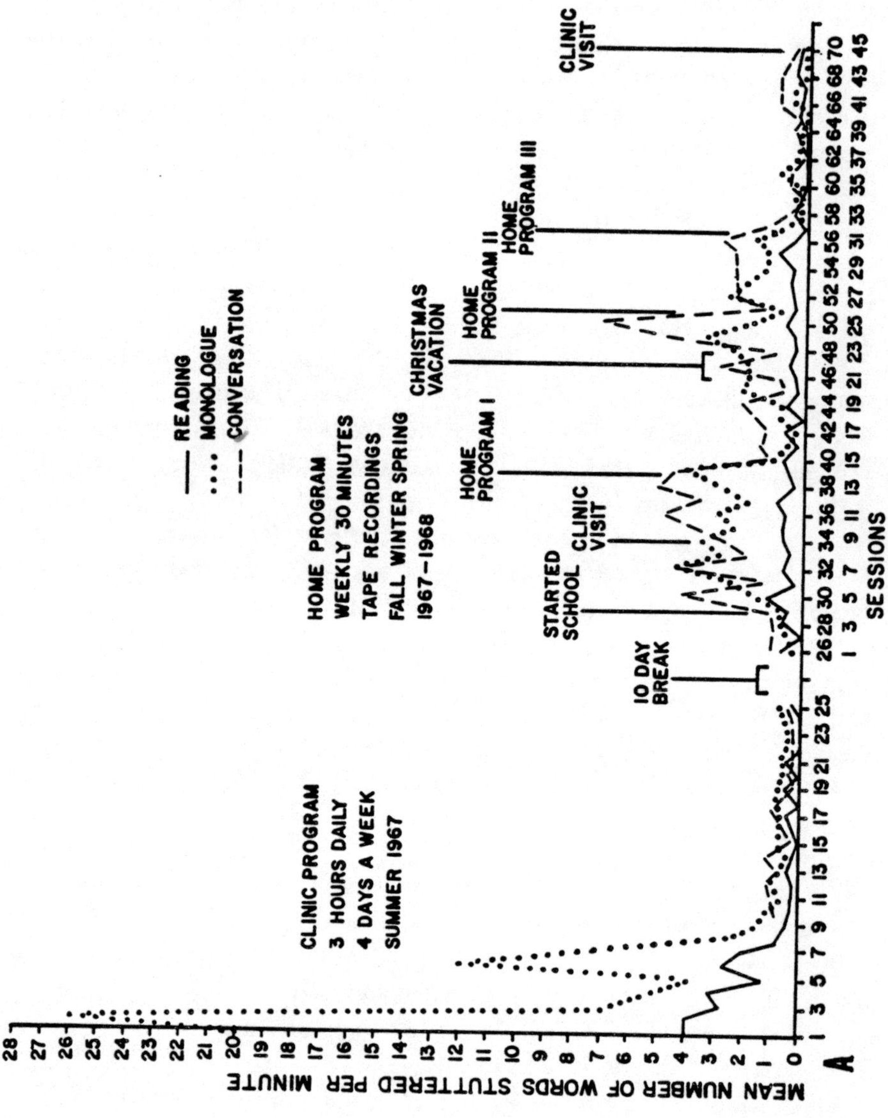
READING
MONOLOGUE
CONVERSATION
CLINIC PROGRAM
3 HOURS DAILY
4 DAYS A WEEK
SUMMER 1967
HOME PROGRAM
WEEKLY 30 MINUTES
TAPE RECORDINGS
FALL WINTER SPRING
1967–1968
10 DAY BREAK
STARTED SCHOOL
CLINIC VISIT
HOME PROGRAM I
CHRISTMAS VACATION
HOME PROGRAM II
HOME PROGRAM III
CLINIC VISIT
MEAN NUMBER OF WORDS STUTTERED PER MINUTE
SESSIONS
A

Figure 22a

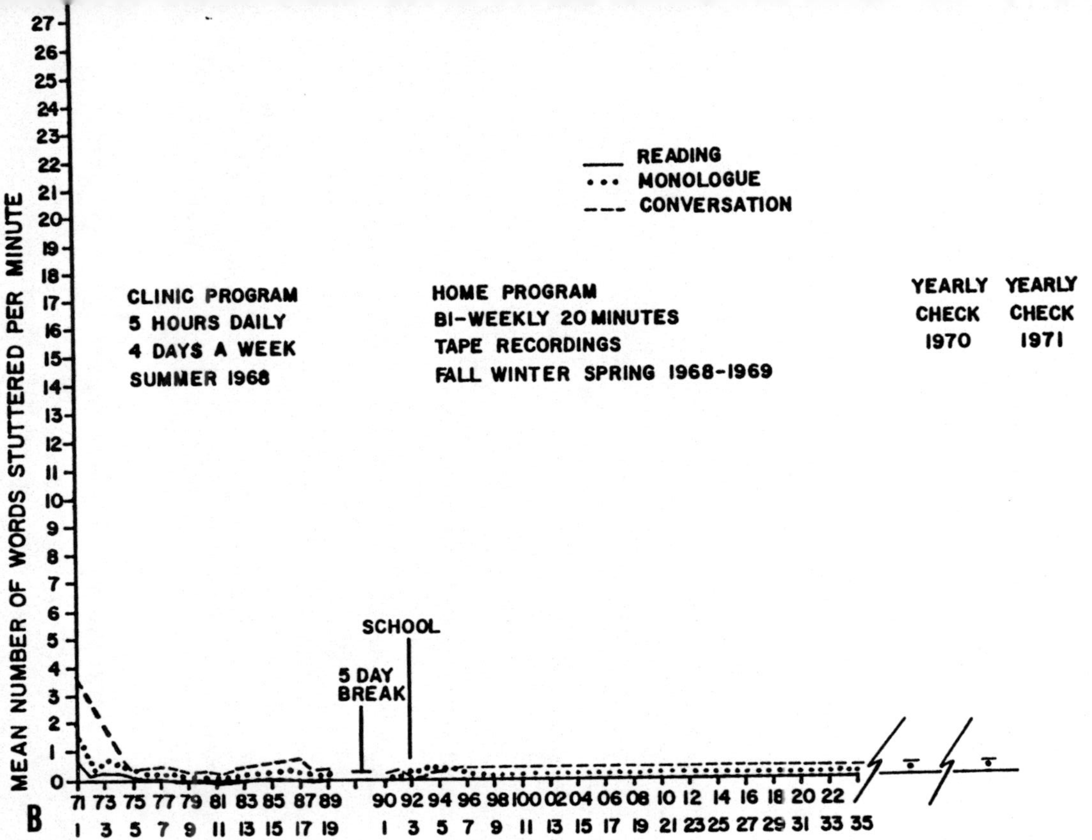

Figure 22b

Figure 22. Means of the number of words stuttered per minute for client SS during clinic and home programs to establish, transfer and maintain fluent reading, monologue and conversation using Program 1, Programmed Traditional.

ification. Stan was to count his stuttered words during the tape recorded sessions. This started in session 39. A decrease in frequency was observed following this modification.

Another gradual increase in frequency was then observed and Home Program Modification II was instituted in session 51. This was the same program with the addition of having Stan replay his tape recordings and count stuttered words from the tape recordings. We had observed that there was an important relationship between his ability to identify stuttered words accurately and his stuttering rate. Again, a decrease in stuttering rate was observed.

Following this, still another increase in frequency of stuttering occurred. Home Program Modification III was then instituted in session 57. A new instruction was added to the program. Stan was to keep reading and talking until he had obtained five consecutive minutes of fluent utterances in each of the modes of reading, monologue and conversation. This again produced a decrease in the frequency of stuttering.

We had been concerned all year about the relationship of his speech performance on the tape recordings to his performance in more natural situations. Both he and his parents had reported that he was generally much more fluent during the tape recording sessions than he was in other situations. He also had demonstrated increased stuttering in special, difficult speaking situations, such as leading prayers at church.

Because of this report we decided to work with him again in the summer of 1968. We replicated the program of the previous summer. We saw him for nineteen sessions, five hours a day with five different clinicians. He did extremely well and commonly operated at less than .5 SW/M.

He then went through another Maintenance Program composed of: 1) bi-weekly tape recordings of monologue and conversation, 2) bi-weekly meetings with his local speech clinician, weekly telephone calls from us and 3) occasional visits to the university clinic. As can be seen in sessions 90 to 122 he continued to maintain his fluency. He continued on the debate squad and placed quite high in many debates.

During 1970 and 1971 we put Stan on a simple Maintenance

Program of yearly postcards and tape recordings. He has continued to maintain his fluency to date. Stan is presently in college and views himself as a normal speaker who occasionally has minor repetitions when he is fatigued. He is studying to be a minister.

We spent 225 hours in therapy with Stan, but this is to be expected during the development of prototypes. Our present programs run much faster (ten to twenty hours) with equal effectiveness. Stan's performance also suggested the need for and the power of Transfer and Maintenance Programs, especially the latter. Finally, Stan demonstrated to us that normal fluency is a reasonable target behavior for people who stutter. Stan was a pioneer client for us in fluency training and we thank him.

Program 2, Delayed Auditory Feedback, Don (DS)

We selected Don as our client illustration of the Delayed Auditory Feedback Program 2 because his program included some special procedures; he went through extremely short sessions, he timed his daily talking and he counted his stuttered words each day.

Don was twenty-one years of age when he came for the initial evaluation. He was an Army student at the Defense Language Institute in Monterey studying Russian and flunking. His Base Rate (Criterion Test) was 10.0 SW/M in reading, 5.0 SW/M in monologue, and 11.4 SW/M in conversation. These were part-word repetitions, whole word repetitions, prolongations and struggle behavior. The Base Rate (Criterion Test) data along with other data are shown in Figure 23. We used a 6-cycle chart from Lindsley (1968) because we wanted to track several events on a daily basis; his count of stuttered words in his environment, his count in daily home practice and his stuttering rate in the clinic sessions. We were also interested in exploring the rate from 0 to 1 SW/M.

He was put through Program 2, Delayed Auditory Feedback, with a criterion level of two minutes at 0 SW/M. Consequently, he took only 2.1 hours of talking time to complete the thirty-step Establishment Program. The actual therapy time including the SI and Criterion Tests took six hours. He operated in the pro-

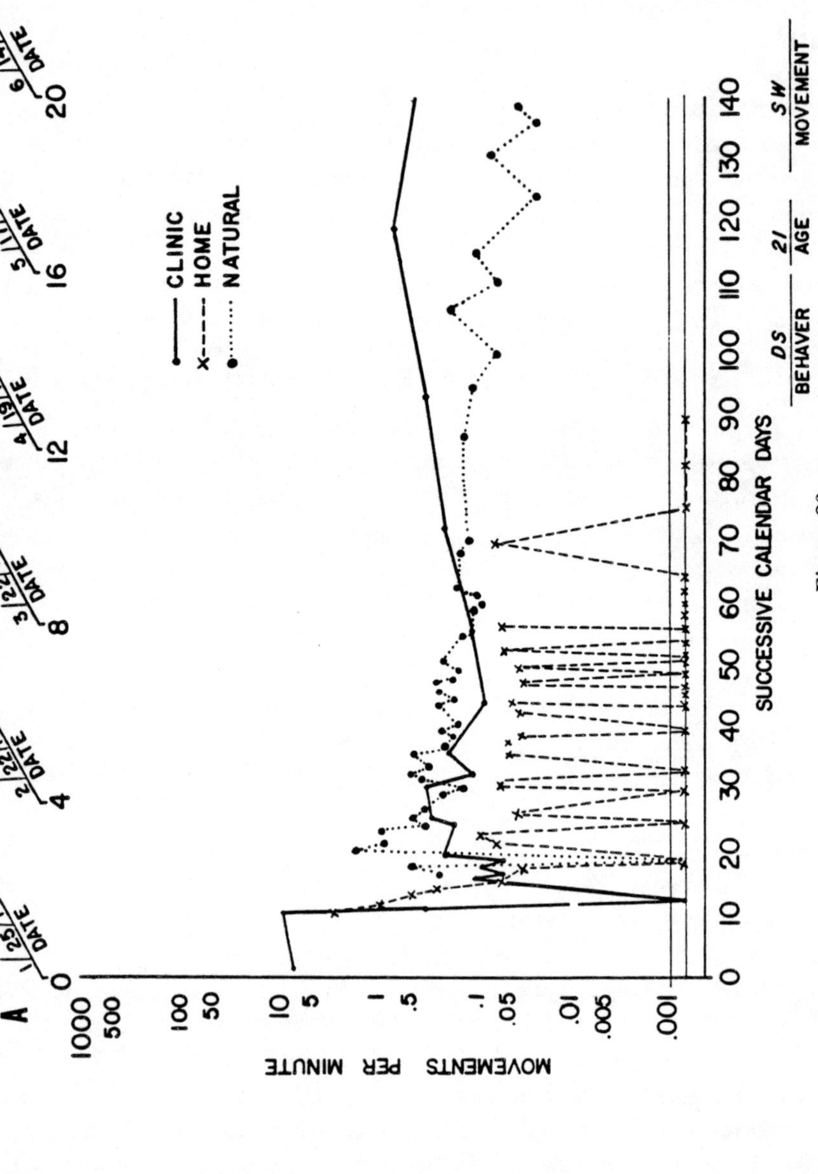
A
MOVEMENTS PER MINUTE
1000
500
100
50
10
5
1
.5
.1
.05
.01
.005
.001
0
1/25/70 DATE
4
2/22/70 DATE
8
3/22/70 DATE
12
4/19/70 DATE
16
5/17/70 DATE
20
6/14/70 DATE
CLINIC
HOME
NATURAL
0 10 20 30 40 50 60 70 80 90 100 110 120 130 140
SUCCESSIVE CALENDAR DAYS
DS
BEHAVER
21
AGE
SW
MOVEMENT

Figure 23a

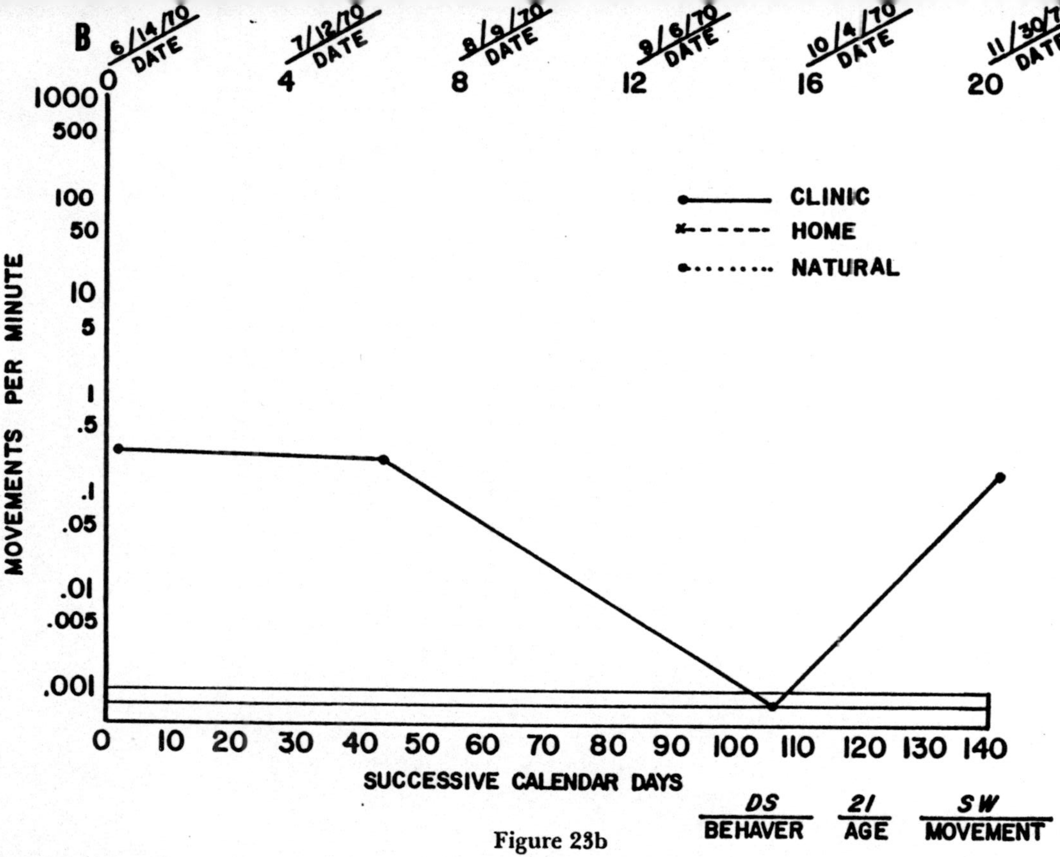

Figure 23b

Figure 23. Means of the number of words stuttered per minute for client DS during clinic, home, and natural environment programs to establish, transfer and maintain fluent reading, monologue and conversation using Program 2, Delayed Auditory Feedback (DAF).

gram at .1 SW/M in both Russian and English. We instituted home practice periods on the first day of therapy. It can be seen in Figure 23 that these generally paralleled his performance at the clinic although initially the SW/M rate at home was higher than in the clinic and later it was lower.

We then began the Transfer Program which included different physical settings, strangers, audience increase and the telephone. We also instituted a count of stuttered words by him in his natural environment. He felt that it was too much to ask him to both count and time his talking with a stopwatch every day so we compromised and let him count stuttered words weekly, but he had to time his talking daily. His talking time averaged two hours a day including weekend days. We used this time as our time base and had him count stuttered words only with a wrist counter to achieve the rest of the environment count data. He found this task onerous, but turned in data on it on a schedule which gradually faded out the counting process. He then was moved into a final sixteen-hour transfer series in which he had to achieve one complete day of fluency. He spent a total of fifty-six minutes talking in the Transfer Program (not including talking in the environment during the natural environment count activity) spread over 3.5 hours of therapy in five sessions. He averaged .1 SW/M in all forms of transfer activities. He engaged in 12.6 hours of home practice in reading, monologue and conversation spread over thirty-five sessions. We gradually faded out the number and duration of home practice periods. His rate during home practice was an average of .01 SW/M.

He was then put on the Maintenance Program which consisted of short periodic clinic visits to collect samples of his reading, monologue and conversation and his report of his SW/M rate in natural situations. We gradually faded these out also. He completed the sixteen-hour transfer step after some minor difficulty. It took him three weeks. He was on the Maintenance Program at the same time. During this same period an interesting event occurred. He reported that when he went home for a one-week vacation he began to stutter again. He took this as a cue to go into a *home practice* routine which he did in the shower on the first day. He came out of the shower and *home practice* and spent the next six days of his vacation speaking fluently with his family. The Maintenance Program included 2.6 hours of his talking, five hours of therapy time and nine sessions. He demonstrated a rate of .2 SW/M (these were commonly whole word repetitions) at the last clinic check some ten months after the conclusion of the Transfer Program proper.

We spent a total of 14.5 hours of therapy with him in nineteen sessions spread out over an eleven-month period. As further proof of his new fluency he graduated near the top of his class in Russian and we received a special phone call and personal commendation from the Commanding Officer at the Defense Language Institute.

Don taught us that the program could be shortened with little or no loss in effectiveness. We did find it necessary, however, to engage in more review steps than is usually necessary when the criterion time is set at a five or ten minute level. Although Don demonstrated normal fluency, he still thought of himself as a stutterer. Follow-up indicated an additional six months of fluency before a gradual relapse over the next three years.

Program 3, Punishment, Dave (DC)

Dave was a fifteen-year-old high school student who was self-referred. He demonstrated whole word repetitions, part-word repetitions, prolongations and broken words (struggle) behavior. His Base Rate (Criterion Test) averaged over three sessions was 10.5 SW/M in monologue and 12.9 SW/M in conversation. We did not take a Base Rate in reading because he did not engage in reading aloud very often and he could only come for two 30-minute sessions weekly. We took one additional Base Rate in front of a video tape recording team and this was 17.0 SW/M in monologue and 16.9 SW/M in conversation. The presence of the recording equipment and personnel served to increase the SW/M rate. The data for these sessions and the rest of the program are shown in Figure 24. We used a straight linear chart for Dave's data.

We also video-taped the first program session (session 5), because we wanted to have a visual record of the effects of the Punishment Program 3. The program consisted basically of the

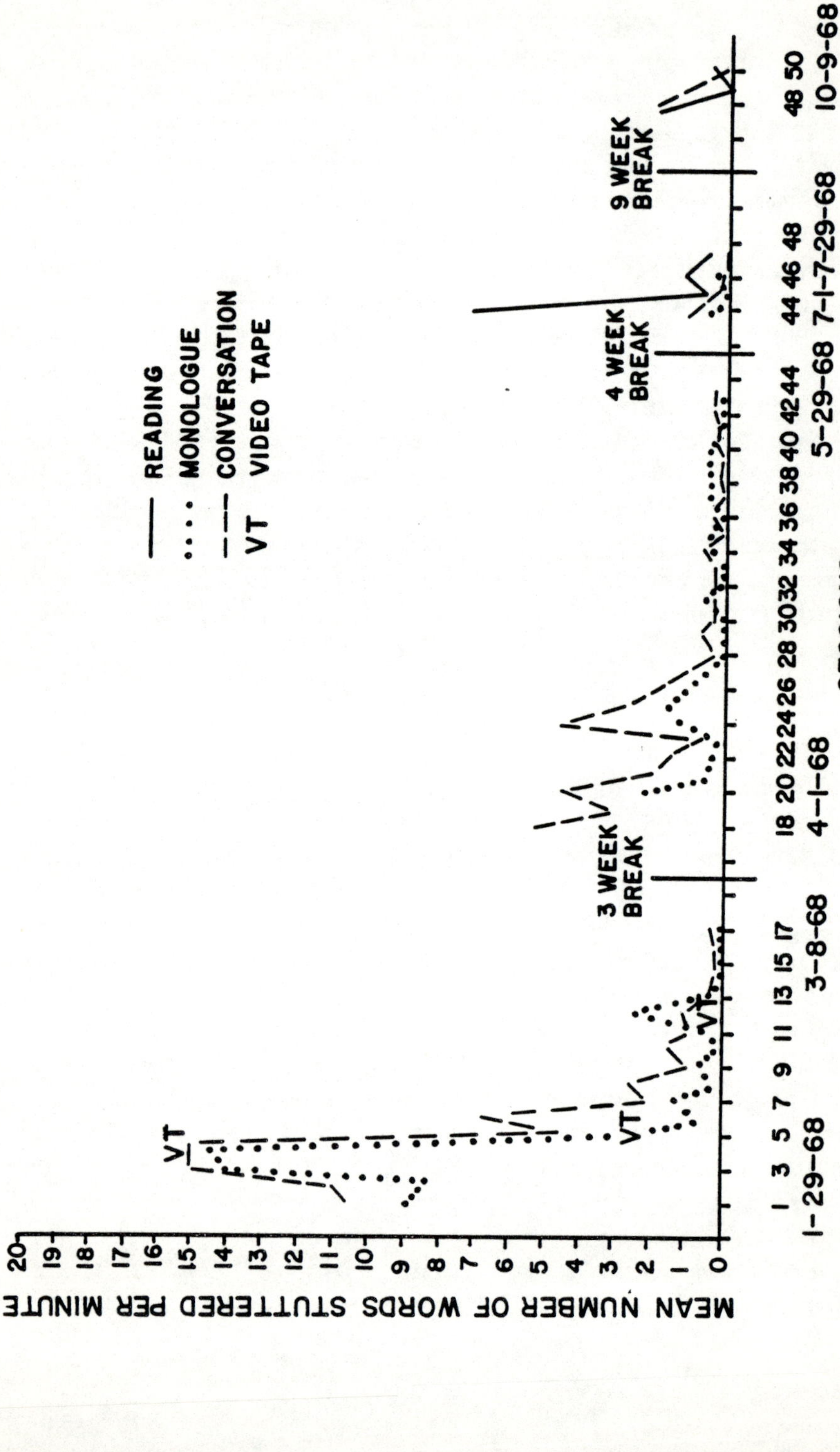

Figure 24. Means of the number of words stuttered per minute for client DC during clinic program to establish, transfer and maintain fluent reading, monologue and conversation using Program 3, Punishment.

clinician defining the four types of stuttered words listed above and saying, "No!," contingently upon the occurrence of each stuttered word. This was our first punishment program and we were all apprehensive about the outcome. During the first thirty minutes of the program (fifteen minutes in monologue and fifteen minutes in conversation) his rate dropped to 3.2 SW/M in monologue and 4.4 SW/M in conversation. His rate continued to drop throughout the next six sessions. We brought him back to the video tape recording studio again for session 12. His rate increased slightly during the taping to 2.5 SW/M in monologue and 1.1 SW/M in conversation. We repeated the Base Rate (Criterion Test) in session 17 and observed .1 SW/M in monologue and .7 SW/M in conversation. This was after 7.3 hours of his talking in seventeen sessions or 11.3 hours of therapy. The effects of punishment on the frequency of stuttering were aptly demonstrated. However, we also observed that there was also much accidental or incidental positive reinforcement of fluency during many of the sessions when the clinician would naturally smile at and joke with Dave while he was fluent.

As part of our procedure at the time we were running Dave, we took a new Base Rate measure each quarter. Dave began therapy again with a new clinician the next quarter. During the Base Rate procedure he demonstrated a rate of 5.3 SW/M in conversation with the new clinician in session 18 and 2.3 SW/M in monologue in session 20. His rate had increased over the three-week break. We continued Base Rate procedures until session 28 because of the fluctuation. We discovered that the new clinician, although instructed only to do Base Rate procedures, had told Dave at the end of each session how many stuttered words he had emitted during the session. He had asked for this information and she felt obliged to give it to him. Our observation was that this procedure was sufficient to continue his new low rate of stuttering and we did not change it. We gradually expanded his talking experiences into several transfer activities of different physical settings, increased audiences and strangers during sessions 30 to 44. His new low rate persisted into transfer activities and he reported that it was carrying over to his speech in other talking situations in life. We involved his friends in the program and asked them to remind him when he stuttered. He ended this quarter in session 43 with a rate of .2 SW/M in conversation and .1 SW/M in monologue.

There was a four-week break and we again changed clinicians and took a new Base Rate measure. Although his monologue remained at .3 SW/M and his conversation at .8 SW/M, his rate in reading (a new mode for him) was 7.3 SW/M. Evidently his fluency in monologue and conversation did not transfer to reading. We solved this by instructing him to read the way he talked i.e. fluently. This instruction alone was enough to bring the rate in reading down to an average of .5 SW/M for the three sessions that we saw him during the summer.

There was a nine-week break before we saw him again. Another new clinician and Base Rate measure indicated 2.0 SW/M in reading and 2.0 SW/M in conversation. With just a frown administered contingently upon stuttered words, the clinician was able to reduce his rate to 0 SW/M in conversation and .2 SW/M in reading.

Because Dave was leaving the area very soon we made one final video tape. His overall rate was less than that of his two nonstuttering friends who made the tape with him. During the tape we asked Dave about his impression of the "No" program. He responded that he found it only slightly irritating initially but that generally it had been very helpful, even when his friends reminded him in other speaking situations. Both Dave and his friends agreed he had improved a great deal in other speaking situations. Unfortunately, we were never able to observe him in his school or other social settings because he would not give us permission to do so.

We were in therapy for fifty sessions or about 33.3 hours of therapy. Our transfer and maintenance procedures were rather casual. Unfortunately, we do not have any additional follow-up data on Dave.

The experience with Dave in this program convinced us that it was indeed, powerful. We were also pleasantly surprised that Dave, himself, viewed the program as a generally positive experience. And well he might because in most of the sessions he was fluent and commonly received only general social approval and incidental, nonprogrammed positive social reinforcement for his fluency.

Program 4, Gradual Increase in Length and Complexity of Utterance, Brian (BH)

The following client was first reported in the *Journal of Speech and Hearing Disorders* (Ryan, 1971). Brian was a nine-year-old male whom we had seen for several diagnostic evaluations for eighteen months previous to instituting this program. His parents were counselled to speak slowly around him, decrease conflicts in the home, etc. He also had received nine months of daily speech therapy in a small group in his school. None of these activities eliminated the stuttering behavior, although there was a reduction from an initial rate of 16.6 SW/M on the SI to 9.6 SW/M. His Base Rate (Criterion Test) before the program was 4.0 SW/M in reading, 9.5 SW/M in monologue and 15.0 SW/M in conversation. His stuttering consisted mostly of part-word repetitions and prolongations. Because the family was moving from the state in a few months, it was decided to engage in a crash program[1] to eliminate his stuttering. The parents brought him to the university clinic on Saturday mornings for three-hour sessions. They also engaged in a daily home program for five minutes a day which paralleled the clinic program. His school speech clinician also carried out a similar program in his school daily. Points were used as reinforcers for fluent utterances. These could be exchanged for toys. For each stuttered word a point was substracted and Brian was required to repeat each stuttered word fluently. His specific program was a variation of GILCU in that a punishment procedure, response cost, was added. Nine different speech clinicians carried out the program, two different ones for each session. The schedule of reinforcement was gradually changed as Brian went through the program. Initially he received a point for thirty seconds of fluency which was given with social reinforcers such as "good" and "fine." The schedule was gradually changed until a point was given only for each five minutes of fluent utterance. Branch steps were devised when Brian demon-

[1] The author wishes to acknowledge the efforts of Barbara Van Kirk in preparing the program and scheduling the various clinicians.

strated that he could not think of anything to talk about and became upset in the clinic session. The branch steps consisted of sixteen steps which started with one fluent word and progressed to 150 seconds of fluent talking (GILCU, Program 4) at which point Brian was put back in the regular sequence. He was reinforced for each correct step in the branch sequence with a point.

The home and school programs carried out each week were important parts of the Transfer Program. In addition, another part of the Transfer Program which involved the entire family was initiated after Brian had completed the conversation mode. This program is shown elsewhere (Ryan, 1971). It provided for Brian's entire family of father, mother, sister and brother to be gradually involved in speaking situations with him.

To provide for maintenance of fluency, the parents were instructed to continue giving Brian points for fluent utterances until he earned enough for a bicycle he wanted. These points were so arranged that he could earn only a maximum number per day, which would permit a gradual accumulation of points to coincide with his birthday some four months after the last session. Brian also sent in weekly postcards from his new home reporting on his fluency and listing the points he had earned for the week.

The results of the program are shown in Figure 25. The immediate reduction in stuttering behavior can be seen in session 1 which worked through reading and started monologue. It was possible to review reading, finish monologue and start conversation in session 2. In session 3, reading and monologue were reviewed and conversation was completed. In session 4 all three modes were reviewed and the Transfer Program begun. In session 5 the Transfer Program was completed. Brian came in one final Saturday two weeks after session 5. His parents were checked on the Maintenance Program and the SI was readministered to Brian. He demonstrated 0.0 SW/M. The amazing, rapid reduction in stuttering both in and out of the clinic during this fifteen-hour program was undoubtedly due partly to excellent home and school cooperation and concurrent home and school programs. The home program involved twenty-four sessions of reading, monologue and conversation for a total of 2.6 hours of

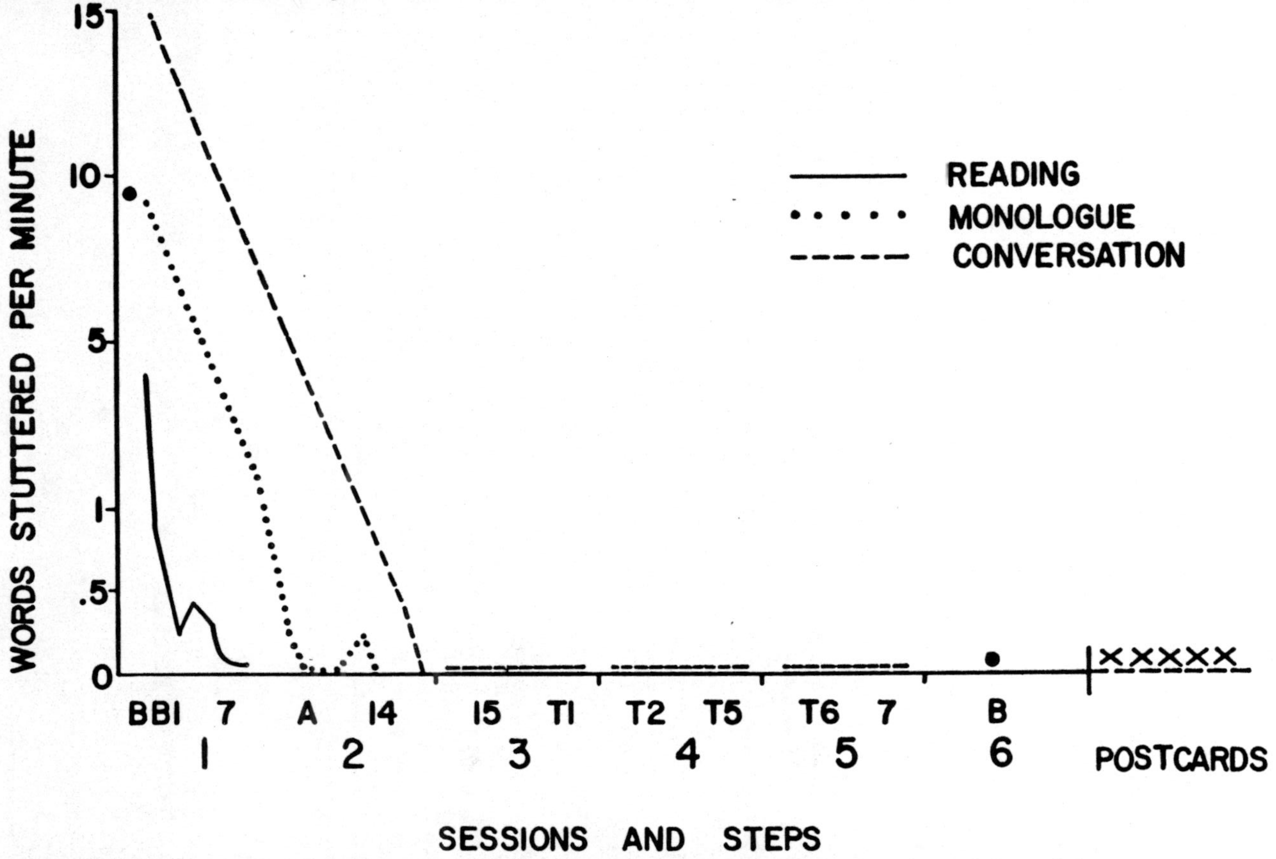

Figure 25. Means of the number of words stuttered per minute for client BH during clinic and home programs to establish, transfer and maintain fluent reading, monologue and conversation using Program 4, Gradual Increase in Length and Complexity of Utterance (GILCU).

Brian's talking. His rate during this home program was .01 SW/M.

Observation in Brian's classroom revealed a similar decrease in stuttering. Postcards sent in by Brian and his parents for three months after the clinic program was completed, reported a continued low rate. A letter from the parents received six months after the conclusion of the clinic program stated that Brian was doing well although he had slipped a little since receiving his bicycle. A tape recording received twelve months later indicated that he was speaking at less than 0.5 SW/M. His parents reported that they occasionally practiced reading, monologue and conversation with him. They also stated that none of his new teachers had noticed any stuttering at school. During a telephone conversation with Brian six months later, he demonstrated a rate of 0.0 SW/M for a 3.5-minute period.

Our experience with Brian taught us several things. The first was that an all-out concentrated effort with concurrent clinic, home and school speech therapy programs was a very powerful way to deal with the problem. We also learned the value of literally *training* parents in the process of therapy, i.e. defining and counting stuttered words and providing appropriate consequences for fluency. His performance with nine different clinicians indicated that it was indeed the program procedure and not the personality of the clinician which resulted in improved fluency. We seemed to achieve instant rapport with "My name is Barbara Van Kirk. I'm your speech clinician for this period. I have the tokens." Of final interest is the observation that during the eighteen-month period following the end of the clinic program proper the parents knew what to do when Brian showed any signs of recurring difficulty. They did some home practice. This is very similar to what Don in Program 2 did on his home visit.

CLIENT PERFORMANCE IN UNUSUAL PROGRAMS

This section is devoted to showing three of the somewhat unusual programs which we carried out only once. The first occurred in the pre-program period with three clients in a study of the prototype of Program 1, Programmed Traditional. It is an abstract of the dissertation by Ryan (1964). The second is a study of the effects of positive reinforcement on stuttering (Ryan, 1967). The third concerns the control of stuttering behavior in a natural setting (Griffin and Van Kirk, 1969). Each of these was presented as a convention paper and they are produced here in entirety with only minor editing.

THE CONSTRUCTION AND EVALUATION OF A PROGRAM FOR MODIFYING STUTTERING BEHAVIOR EMPLOYING OPERANT CONDITIONING PRINCIPLES

PURPOSE

The purpose of this study was to construct and evaluate a program for modifying stuttering behavior in oral reading utilizing responses suggested by Van Riper's cancellation therapy (1963) and appropriate response-reinforcement contingencies, i.e. Van Riper's procedures were programmed.

METHOD

Subjects

The subjects were three stutterers who had never received speech therapy and who stuttered when they read aloud. They were 16, 42, and 23 years of age, respectively. They were paid $2.00 per session for participating in the study.

The Program

An eight-step program, modelled after Van Riper (1963), consisted of the following steps while the subject was reading aloud continuously changing reading material: 1) *experimenter identification,* in which the experimenter signalled the subject during and/or after each stuttered word; 2) *experimenter-subject identi-*

Note: Reprinted by permission of the authors; Bruce Ryan, and George Shames, Professor of Speech, the University of Pittsburgh. This paper was presented at the annual convention of the American Speech and Hearing Association in November in Washington, D.C., 1966.

fication, in which the subject and the experimenter concurrently signalled when they observed a stuttered word; 3) *cancellation*$_1$, in which the subject reiterated stuttered words once; 4) *cancellation*$_2$, in which the subject reiterated a stuttered word in a prolonged manner; 5) *cancellation*$_3$, in which the subject reiterated a stuttered word with a prolongation of the initial sound of the word; 6) *pullout*$_1$, in which the subject interrupted stuttering behavior with a prolongation of the initial sound of the word; 7) *pullout*$_2$, in which the subject interrupted stuttering behavior with a prolongation of the initial sound of the word within a 1.5-second time limit; and 8) *prolongation,* in which the subject initiated a word upon which he anticipated stuttering with a prolongation of the initial sound of the word.

The Response-Reinforcement Contingencies

The subjects were reinforced in a negative reinforcement paradigm, i.e. reading aloud to the experimenter was viewed as an aversive situation, and reductions in reading time were contingent on the subjects emitting the desired behavior appropriate in each of the eight steps of the program. These reductions in reading time were signalled by using an electric clock-counter, numbered one to sixty in full view of both the experimenter and the subjects. The hand of the clock moved to the next number after each correct response. The subjects read in any given trial (one trial each day) until they had emitted sixty correct responses and in any step (one through eight) until they reached at least 75 per cent accuracy (sixty correct responses out of eighty words stuttered). If the subjects failed to reach criterion in three successive trials, they were returned to the previous step. A schedule of continuous, 100 per cent reinforcement was employed.

Equipment and Materials

The subjects read aloud in an I.A.C. booth. A RNT Standard Time Interval Clock (an electric clock), with only a minute hand and a specially constructed face displaying the numbers, one to sixty was placed in the I.A.C. booth to the subject's right and clicked audibly each time the minute hand moved one (minute) marker. A specially constructed clock-control system permitted:

1) the clock to run automatically; or 2) be operated by the experimenter (button A). A Maico, model F-1, audiometer was used to generate a 500 cps tone (not heard by the subjects) which was recorded along with the subject's voice on a Bell RT-75 tape recorder each time the experimenter observed a stuttered word and pressed the appropriate button (button B). The tones were tabulated for counts of frequency of stuttering. All reading sessions were tape recorded for later analysis. An Industrial Timer Controls Timer, model P-4R, made it possible to accurately time the desired behavior in step seven, $pullout_2$. The subjects read from books in the "high interest, low reading level" category.

Definition of Stuttering Behavior

Only stuttered words were counted. The senior author was the sole judge of the occurrence of stuttered words during the program. His accuracy was checked by comparing his judgments of fifteen-minute tape recorded samples of the three subjects' oral reading with those of two other speech pathologists who had considerable experience with the problem of stuttering. Phi correlations were computed and ranged from .79 to .92. This is comparable to reliability ratings in other studies of stuttering behavior (Wingate, 1959).

RESULTS AND DISCUSSION

The Pre-Program Phase

The pre-program stuttering behavior of Subjects One and Two will be discussed in some detail because this behavior represented an incidental finding concerning the operant analysis of stuttering behavior and affected the performance of Subjects One and Two in the program which followed.

Subject One read one hour daily for five days with the clock running automatically supposedly clicking once each minute as it moved to the next minute marker. It can be noted in Figure 26 that the stuttering behavior, expressed in relative frequency (percentage) of words stuttered, of Subject One increased both within and between each of these readings. This observation appeared contrary to previous research of stuttering adaptation (a

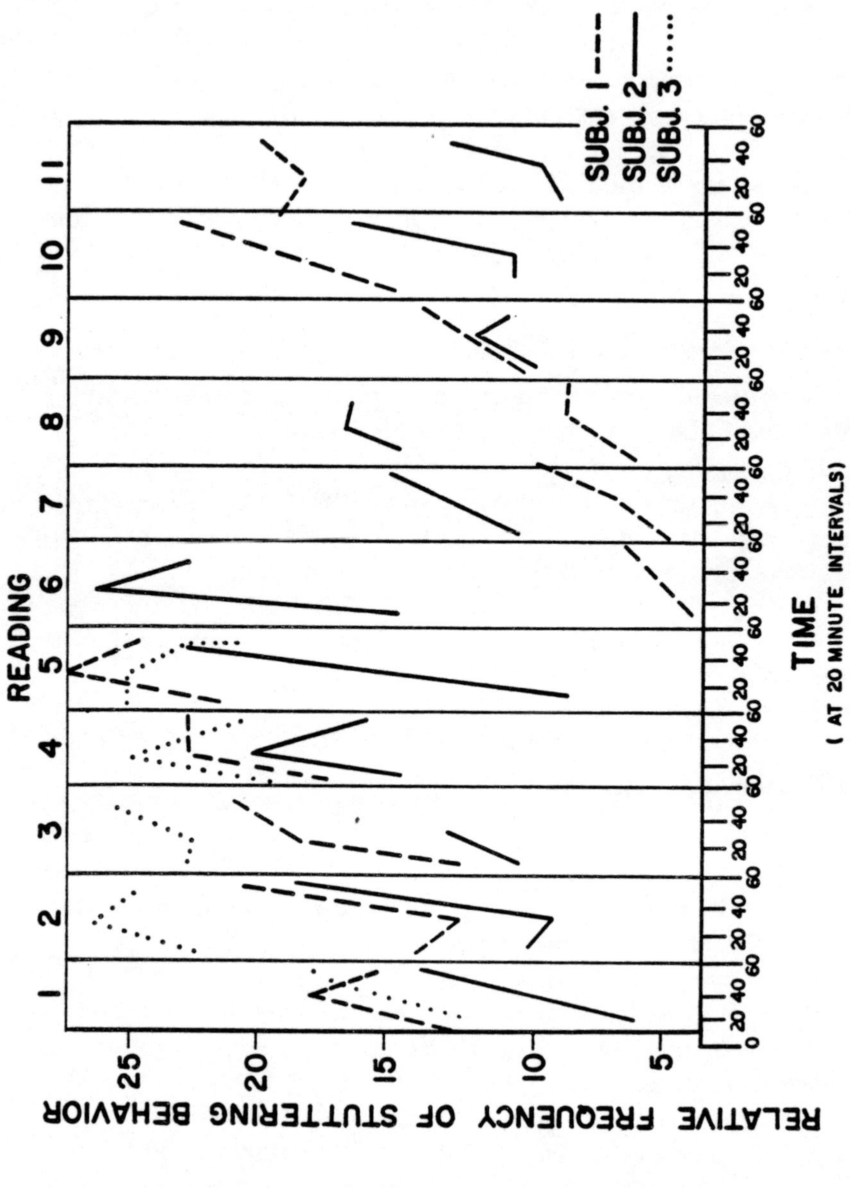

Figure 26. Means of the relative frequency (percentage) of stuttering of three subjects during the pre-program readings.

gradual decrease in the frequency of stuttered words during a reading) within reading sessions of continuously changing reading material (Goldiamond, 1965; Johnson, 1955). The following day, Subject One was started in the program. A sharp decrease in stuttering behavior was observed. This decrease persisted into step two. (These decreases are not shown in Figure 26 but were comparable to those shown in the first minutes of readings 6-8.) Examination of the tape recordings of the first five readings revealed that the recordings varied from fifty to fifty-six minutes instead of being sixty minutes in duration. It was also noted that the clock clicked twice (moved two minute markers) in a number of instances which accounted for the reduced reading time. A technical artifact in the wiring of the clock control system was discovered which had resulted in the extra clicks and movements of the clock. Thus, if button B, used for identifying stuttered words, was depressed at the same time that the clock was automatically moving to the next minute marker, the minute hand would move an extra minute. It was postulated that the stuttering behavior of Subject One had come under the control of the clock clicks during the first five readings. This would account for both the increase in stuttering behavior during these readings and the decrease in stuttering behavior noted during the first two steps in the program. To test this hypothesis, Subject One was asked to read for another five 1-hour daily readings (readings 6-10). During these five readings, the experimenter controlled the clock causing it to click and move at approximately one-minute intervals always immediately following a stuttered word. Occasionally the experimenter caused the minute hand to move twice. This represented a simulation of the conditions of the first five readings. It can be seen in Figure 26, that the stuttering behavior of Subject One gradually increased both within and between these second five readings. His stuttering behavior was under the control of the clock clicking.

Subject Two read for five 1-hour daily readings with the clock running automatically. The technical artifact was discovered after Subject Two had read for three days. Readings 4 and 5 were accomplished with the clock running automatically, but the technical artifact removed. It can be seen in Figure 26 that Subject Two demonstrated a gradual increase in stuttering behavior both between and within readings with the exception of reading 4, the first reading in which the technical artifact was not present. It appeared that the stuttering behavior of Subject Two had also come under the control of the clock clicking. To test this hypothesis, reading 6 was conducted with the experimenter controlling the clock and causing it to click immediately after stuttered words at approximately one-minute intervals and occasionally to click twice. It can be noted that the stuttering behavior of Subject Two reached a new high frequency in this reading. As an alternative method of testing the original hypothesis the next four readings (7-10) were accomplished with the experimenter controlling the clock and attempting to cause it to click only after fluent words. As can be seen in Figure 26, the stuttering behavior of Subject Two during readings 7 to 10 continued to demonstrate an increase within readings but a gradual decrease of stuttering between readings, especially between reading 6 and readings 7 to 10. It was concluded that the stuttering behavior of Subject Two had also come under the control of the clock clicking during the first three readings. His stuttering behavior increased or decreased contingent upon the presentation of clock clicks after stuttered or fluent words.

Subject Three read for five 1-hour daily readings with the clock not operating.

The Base Operant Level Phase

To determine the base operant level of stuttering behavior and program operant behavior of Subjects One and Two, they were asked to read aloud in their normal manner for an hour with no clock clicking (reading 11). Reading 5 was used for Subject Three.

The Program Phase

An analysis of the program operant behavior of the three subjects during the base and final operant level readings and the program is shown in Table XV. Generally, these were the behaviors which were to be taught during the program and by definition oc-

TABLE XV

ANALYSIS OF PROGRAM OPERANT BEHAVIOR

	Program Steps								Total	
Subjects and Measures	*1*	*2*	*3*	*4*	*5*	*6*	*7*	*8*	*Total*	*Total Means*
Subject 1										
Base operant level	*	*	1.7%	.6%	0.0%	0.0%	*	.9%	3.2%	
Program										
Mean	100.0%	61.5%	79.7%	70.3%	74.2%	84.5%	83.5%	90.1%		69.2%
Number trials	3	7	1	3	2	1	2	2		2.6
Final operant level	*	*	0.0%	0.0%	1.4%	0.0%	*	13.9%	15.3%	
Subject 2										
Base operant level	*	*	.7%	0.0%	.1%	0.0%	*	11.8%	12.6%	
Program										
Mean	100.0%	52.5%	76.1%	74.5%	80.4%	81.3%	75.8%	68.7%		64.9%
Number trials	2	4	1	4	1	1	1	4		2.0
Final operant level	*	*	0.0%	0.0%	2.8%	0.0%	*	11.1%	13.9%	
Subject 3										
Base operant level	*	*	1.0%	.4%	0.0%	.5%	*	20.8%	22.7%	
Program										
Mean	100.0%	85.3%	98.4%	80.1%	91.2%	78.9%	76.0%	71.5%		83.9%
Number trials	1	3	1	1	1	1	2	2		1.5
Final operant level	*	*	.4%	0.0%	0.0%	.5%	*	43.9%	44.8%	
Additional reading	*	*	0.0%	0.0%	0.0%	3.3%	*	79.6%	82.9%	

* Not measured.

curred concurrently with stuttering operants. The program operant, prolongation of the initial sound of a word, was also classified as a stuttering operant. The frequency of these behaviors is expressed as a percentage representing the ratio of program operants to stuttering operants. Step one, experimenter identification; step two, experimenter-subject identification; and step seven, $pullout_2$ were not measured during the base operant level reading due to the nature of these steps. It was noted that the program operant behavior of Subject One was at relatively low strength and consisted of only 3.2 per cent of his stuttering behavior. The program operant behavior of Subject Two was at somewhat higher strength but still constituted only 12.6 per cent of his stuttering behavior. Subject Three demonstrated 22.7 per cent program operant behavior, the highest of the three subjects.

There were basically two response classes required in the program: 1) the detection of stuttered words and 2) the emission of appropriate modification responses. The subjects experienced difficulty in either or both of these areas. The attenuated stuttering behavior of all three of the subjects during the program contributed to their difficulty with the emission of the first response class, detection.

Subjects One and Two achieved means of 69.2 per cent and 64 per cent accuracy, respectively, for the entire program. They required a mean of 2.6 and 2.0 trials per step, respectively, to complete the program. They required 20.9 and 20.1 hours, respectively, to complete the eight-step program. In contrast, Subject Three achieved a mean of 73.9 per cent accuracy, needed only a mean of 1.5 trials per step and spent only 3.3 hours in the eight-step program. Step Two appeared to be the most difficult for all three subjects. The differences in these performances were due to the attenuated stuttering behavior of Subjects One and Two. Subject Three became progressively less accurate in steps five through eight (a range of means of 91.2 per cent to 71.5 per cent).

All three subjects demonstrated generalization of program operants to the final operant level reading. Subject One demonstrated an increase to 15.3 per cent program operant behavior over his base percentage of 3.2 per cent. The greatest increase was in prolongation of the initial sound (13.9 per cent), the end-goal response taught in the program.

Subject Two demonstrated a total of 13.9 per cent program operant behavior which was only slightly greater than his base level (12.6 per cent). The percentage of prolongation operants remained about the same (11.8 per cent vs. 11.1 per cent). There was a slight increase in pullout$_1$ behavior from .1 per cent to 2.8 per cent.

Subject Three demonstrated an increase in program operant behavior from 22.7 per cent in the base operant level reading to 44.8 per cent in the final operant level reading (43.9 per cent was prolongation behavior). This behavior was so different from his previous reading in step eight that he was asked to read again and given instructions to prolong initial sounds (the same instructions as in step eight). No other response-reinforcement contingencies were presented. During this additional reading he demonstrated 82.9 per cent program operant behavior composed of 79.6 per cent prolongation behavior and 3.3 per cent pullout behavior. Instructions had become important discriminative stimuli for the program operant behavior of Subject Three.

Stuttering Operants

The relative frequency (percentage) of stuttering behavior during the base and final operant level readings and the program readings for all three subjects is shown in Figure 27. During the base level reading Subject One demonstrated a relative frequency of 17.6 per cent which was derived from a stuttering rate of 11.6 words stuttered per minute and a reading rate of 62.5 words read per minute. Subject Two demonstrated 10.3 per cent stuttering behavior which represented a stuttering rate of 11.9 words stuttered per minute and a reading rate of 115.3 words read per minute. Subject Three demonstrated a relative frequency of stuttering behavior of 24 per cent which represented his stuttering rate of 16.8 words stuttered per minute and reading rate of 69.6 words read per minute.

Subjects One and Two demonstrated immediate sharp decreases in stuttering behavior upon entering the program in step one.

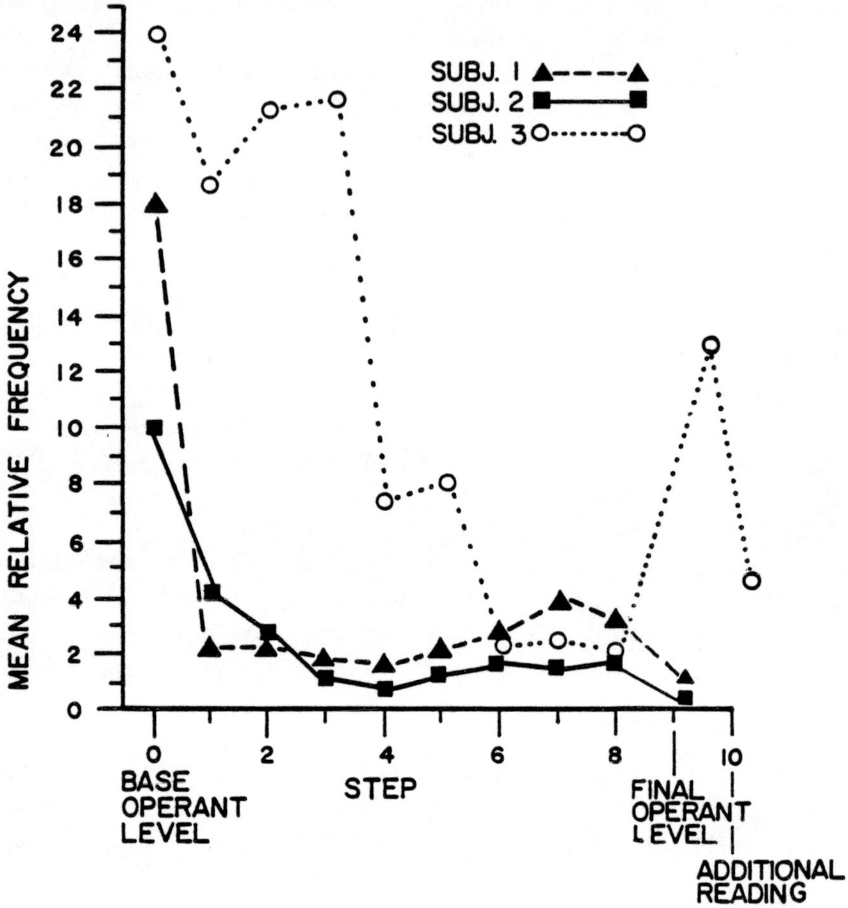

Figure 27. Means of the relative frequency (percentage) of stuttering of three subjects during the Eight-Step Program and the base and final operant level readings.

Subject Three by contrast demonstrated a relatively gradual decrease in stuttering behavior except for the great decrease from step three to step four. This may have been due to an interaction between prolongation behavior which retarded his total word output rate and the incompatibility of cancellation$_2$ behavior and stuttering behavior.

The effects of the program generalized to the post-program

reading. Subject One continued to demonstrate a low relative frequency of stuttering (1.2 per cent derived from a stuttering rate of 1.2 words stuttered per minute and a reading rate of 98.7 words read per minute). Subject Two also continued to demonstrate reduced stuttering behavior (.4 per cent derived from .6 words stuttered per minute and 142.0 words read per minute). Subject Three also demonstrated a reduction in stuttering behavior from the base operant level to the final operant level (13.2 per cent derived from 11.5 words stuttered per minute and 86.6 words read per minute). However, this stuttering behavior differed greatly from his stuttering behavior in step eight (1.1 per cent derived from 1.8 words stuttered per minute and 149.4 words read per minute). In the additional reading he demonstrated 5.5 per cent relative frequency of stuttering behavior derived from 7.1 words stuttered per minute and 133.1 words read per minute.

Generalization to Reading and Speaking Outside the Program

Subjects One and Two reported reading in other situations "very fluently" to others. Subject Three reported that there was no generalization of the effects of the program to any noticeable extent to his reading at home. Casual observation of all three subjects' speech revealed no gross changes in their speaking behavior.

Clinical Implications

The reading program discussed in this study may be viewed as part of a larger program of the modification of stuttering which could include speaking behavior and generalization to common speaking situations. A reading program may be the initial step in the clinical management of stuttering. Goldiamond (1965) suggests this possibility. The eight-step program or a variation of it (perhaps fewer steps would be equally effective) could be employed while the stutterer spoke. Other response-reinforcement contingencies could be used, e.g. social reinforcement on an intermittent schedule. Fluent speaking could supplant fluent reading if the stimuli (printed words) were gradually faded and the stutterer had to speak, spontaneously, to fill the blank spaces between the printed words.

The observation that stuttering behavior which had come under the control of certain reinforcement contingencies decreased sharply when these reinforcement contingencies were altered may have important clinical implications. Furthermore, it may be that increases in stuttering behavior in initial phases and decreases in later phases of common stuttering therapies may somehow be related to or explained by this paradigm. Initially the therapist offers positive reinforcement for stuttering, i.e. he accepts and encourages stuttering behavior. Stuttering behavior increases partially due to the elimination of the stutterer's efforts to hide his stuttering. Later in therapy the therapist introduces modification or other procedures or simply stops reinforcing stuttering behavior. Stuttering behavior decreases, partially due to the effectiveness of the modifications. Further research concerning this paradigm may offer more effective clinical procedures.

THE EFFECTS OF POSITIVE REINFORCEMENT ON THE FREQUENCY OF STUTTERING BEHAVIOR

There are many possible programs for the operant manipulation of stuttering behavior (Flanagan, Goldiamond and Azrin, 1958; Goldiamond, 1965; Rickard and Mundy, 1965; Martin and Siegel, 1966a; 1966b; Leach, 1969; Martin, 1968). Few studies, however, have assessed the effectiveness of positive reinforcement administered contingently upon the emission of stuttered words. Shames and Sherrick (1965) postulated that stuttering, commonly viewed as learned and maintained in a negative reinforcement paradigm, might be brought under the control of a positive reinforcer. Once this control had been established, the removal of the positive reinforcer should result in the elimination of the

Note: Reprinted by permission of the author, Bruce Ryan. This paper was presented at the annual convention of the American Speech and Hearing Association in November in Chicago, 1967.

stuttering. Ryan (1964) observed a similar process. This study, Program 1, explored the Shames-Sherrick hypothesis. The results suggested Program II, which was quite different in both procedure and rationale.

METHOD

Subject

A twelve-year-old male who stuttered served as the single subject. He had been receiving speech therapy prior to participating in this study. Because he had a record of poor attendance and negativism toward speech therapy he was paid $.50 a day for attending the sessions promptly and consistently. He demonstrated perfect attendance.

Procedures

The subject was instructed before each session. He read aloud daily, five days a week, sixty minutes a day from high interest, low reading level books of continuously changing reading material. There were twenty-three readings. All readings were tape recorded. Hand counters were used to count both the number of words stuttered and the number of reinforcers offered. The number of words read per session was counted by pre-counting the words in the reading material and noting the starting and stopping points for each reading.

Base Level

The first five readings (1-5) were to determine the subject's pre-program level or base level of stuttering frequency. He was instructed to read aloud for 60 minutes each day.

Program I

Program I was instituted during the next five readings (6-10). The subject was instructed to read aloud as before. In addition, he was told that he would receive a penny for each click of a hand counter which was then held where he could see it and hear it click. The experimenter clicked the hand counter immediately after each stuttered word. Reinforcement was administered on a 100 per cent continuous schedule. The subject was told at the end of each reading how much he had earned, but he was not paid until the conclusion of the study.

Extinction

For the next five readings (11-15) the subject was given the same instructions as in the previous readings, but the instruction about earning money for clicks was excluded, and the hand counter was removed from the subject's view.

Program II

During the extinction phase in Program I there was an increase in the frequency of stuttering blocks but a reduction in their duration. These results suggested Program II. For the next eight readings (16-23) Program II was instituted. It consisted of re-instructing the subject that he would receive a penny for each click of the counter, similar to Program I. The experimenter, however, differentially reinforced stuttered words. He reinforced only those stuttered words which approximated fluent ones. These were commonly some form of prolongation. Throughout these eight readings progressively shorter prolongations were reinforced. The reinforcement schedule again was 100 per cent.

RESULTS

The results in means of the number of words read per minute and words stuttered per minute for all twenty-three readings are shown in Figure 28.

Base Level

For these five readings the mean of the number of words stuttered per minute was 11.2 and the mean of the number of words read per minute was 63.4. There was variation in stuttering frequency and reading rate during these readings. There was no consistent relationship between reading rate and stuttering rate.

Program I

In reading 6, a decrease in both stuttering rate and reading rate was observed. This was similar to that noted by Wingate (1959), Goldiamond (1965), Martin and Siegel (1966b) and Martin

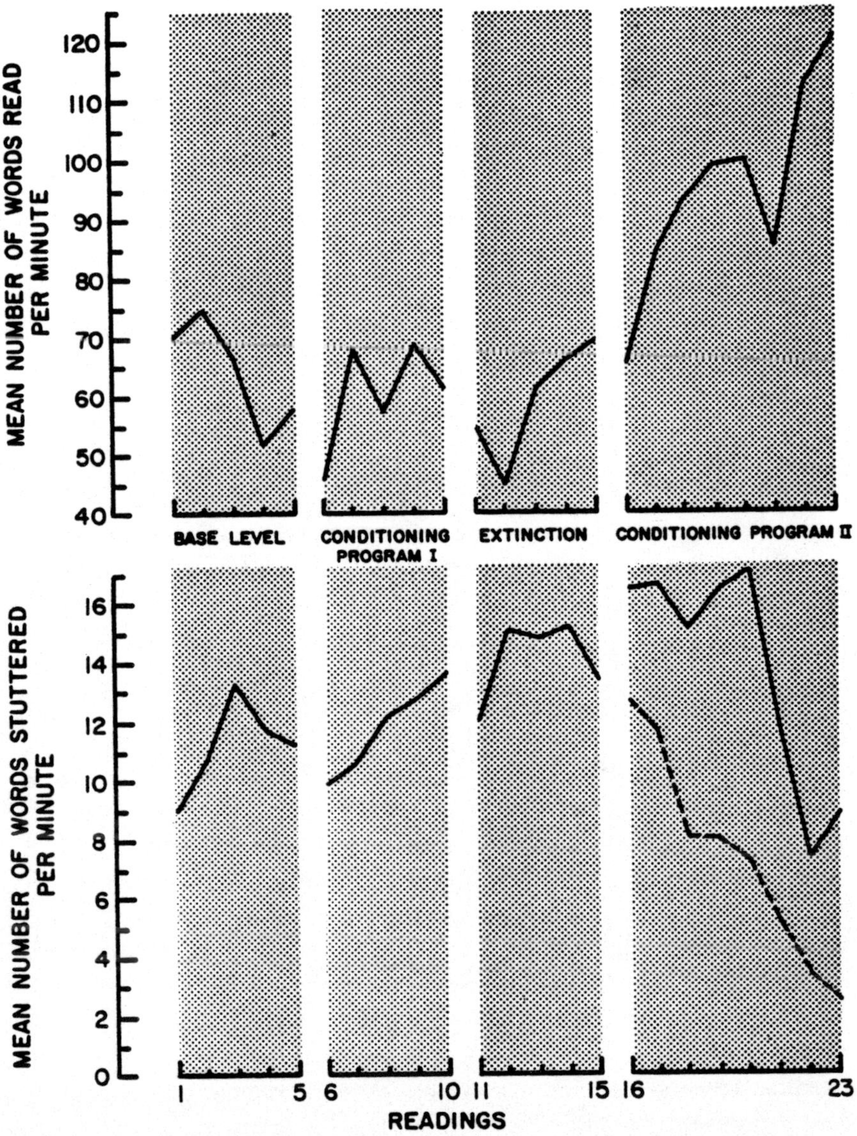

Figure 28. Means of the number of words read per minute and words stuttered per minute by the subject during base level, Conditioning Program I, extinction, and Conditioning Progam II.

(1968) when "attention" is drawn to stuttering behavior. Immediately after reading 6 the subject verbalized the response-reinforcement contingency, i.e. he said, "You clicked that thing each time I stuttered." During this reading the administration of a click contingent upon stuttering behavior had acted as a punishing event. Although the reading rate varied greatly during these five readings (6-10) the frequency of the stutterings gradually increased until it reached a new high of 13.6 words stuttered per minute during reading 10. The click began to function as a positive reinforcer and the stuttering behavior had come under the control of it.

Extinction

During these five readings (11-15) there was a gradual increase in stuttering behavior to 14.1 words stuttered per minute. These data did not support the Shames-Sherrick hypothesis that removal of a positive reinforcer would result in a decrease in stuttering behavior.

Program II

Stuttering rate increased initially during these eight readings (16-23) and then decreased sharply in reading 22 to a new low of 7.0 words stuttered per minute. The solid line in the lower right hand portion of Figure 28 represents the frequency of both *large* stuttered words which were not reinforced and *small* stuttered words which were reinforced. Reading rate increased over these eight readings until it reached a new high of 121.2 words read per minute in reading 23.

The experimenter had observed during Program II that he often had difficulty distinguishing between a fluent word and a short or small stuttered prolongation. The incongruity of almost normal reading rate accompanied by a relatively high stuttering rate suggested the possibility that the experimenter had counted (reinforced) a number of fluent words as stuttered words during these readings. To test this hypothesis, the experimenter waited six months so that he would *forget* the criteria he had used to judge stuttering events during the conditioning periods. He then listened to the eight tape recordings and counted stuttered words again. The results of this analysis are represented by the broken line in the lower right hand portion of Figure 28 and included *large* stuttered words (part-word repetitions and struggle behavior). These data revealed a decrease in stuttering rate to a new low of 2.6 words stuttered per minute in reading 23. This seemed commensurate with the observed increase in reading rate. The experimenter had reinforced and counted a number of fluent words as stuttered words during Program II. This would also explain why the subject read more fluently, i.e. he was gradually reinforced for more and more fluent utterances. A program of successive approximation using differential positive reinforcement of stuttering was effective in the reduction of stuttering behavior.

Reliability

To establish the reliability of the experimenter, twenty 1-minute tape recorded segments were selected from the ten base level and extinction phase readings. The experimenter and an observer independently listened to these recordings and counted stuttered words. The correlation between the count of the experimenter and the observer was .93.

DISCUSSION

Although the data in this study did not support the Shames-Sherrick hypothesis, two methodological problems may cast doubt upon the adequacy of Program I to do so. First, it is possible that adequate control by the positive reinforcer had not been established during the conditioning period, and, second, the length of the extinction phase may not have been long enough to permit extinction. An increase in response frequency is common during the early phases of the extinction process (Skinner, 1953). These methodological inadequacies and the results of the study by Ryan (1964) in which alteration of response-reinforcement contingencies did produce dramatic decreases in stuttering behavior suggest that further study of the Shames-Sherrick hypothesis should be made.

Program II offers another operant procedure which may have value in therapy for stuttering. It is similar to the programs by

Rickard and Mundy (1965) and Leach (1969) in that it established fluent vocalization using positive reinforcement. It was different in that the subject's behavior was gradually shaped from stuttering to fluency in a predetermined manner while he was reading aloud.

This study also raises some methodological questions. When the experimenter is observing gradual changes in behavior it may be very difficult to maintain precise definitions of the desired behavior. This becomes especially important as the subject becomes more fluent and even his *stuttering* responses are small, fluent-like utterances. It was observed in this program that initially an increase in the frequency of stuttering behavior occurred. This may be aversive to both the therapist and the subject. Another problem concerns frequency, the usual criterion measure in operant paradigms. The frequency of stuttering responses may be misleading as it was in this study. Other parameters such as duration, topography and total word output rate may also be important (Goldiamond, 1965). A final problem concerns the end-goal response of any program for eliminating stuttering. The subject in this study demonstrated a final reading rate within normal limits. The stuttering behavior he exhibited was minor in the last few readings. Should the goal in stuttering therapy be normal fluency which contains some disfluencies (Johnson, 1961) or some kind of superfluency with no disfluencies? Perkins (1967) has raised this same question.

The results of this study suggest that Program II has clinical application, if clinicians can devise programs of a sequence of clearly defined behaviors and maintain these definitions as the behaviors gradually change. The findings in this study may also explain the success of traditional therapy approaches which utilize symptom management such as those described by Van Riper (1963) and programmed by Ryan (1964). The phenomenon of the self-recovered stutterer may be due to a process of self-discovered, self-imposed and self-reinforced sequences of successive approximations of fluency.

The operant programs for controlling and/or eliminating stuttering are many. It remains for further research to demonstrate which are most effective.

Author's Note: The recent study by Shaw and Shrum (1972) demonstrated quite conclusively that positive reinforcement could indeed increase the frequency of stuttering behavior.

MODIFICATION OF STUTTERING BEHAVIOR IN A NATURAL ENVIRONMENT

It has been shown that stuttering behavior can be modified using operant technology. Most of these attempts have been within a *laboratory* setting. This report concerns the modification of stuttering behavior within a natural classroom setting.

Subject HW received twenty sessions of therapy for his stuttering at a University Speech and Hearing Center during winter term, 1966. His stuttering responses were shaped toward more fluent responses in a reading and monologue situation. During this time, his speaking rate increased and his stuttering rate greatly decreased. A change was noted in the topography of the stuttered word, namely, that the stuttering blocks were smaller. Fluency was reportedly maintained in several environmental situations immediately following therapy. However, one year later, a recheck in the clinic revealed a stuttering rate of 1.5 SW/M in both reading and speaking. It was also reported that fluency had broken down in the environment. In January, 1969, HW began teaching a class in Educational Psychology. Fourteen students majoring in speech pathology and audiology were enrolled in the class along with thirty-three other students. A baseline measure taken during the second class meeting revealed 5.4 SW/M in the classroom situation consisting of approximately 90 per cent monologue and 10 per cent conversation. These data are presented in Figure 29.

Step one of the program consisted of making HW aware that

Note: Reprinted by permission of the authors; Kathleen Griffin, Director, Speech and Hearing Clinic, Glendale Adventist Hospital, Los Angeles, California, and Barbara Van Kirk, The Easter Seal Society Rehabilitation Center, Bridgeport, Connecticut. This paper was presented at the annual convention of the American Speech and Hearing Association in November in Chicago, 1969.

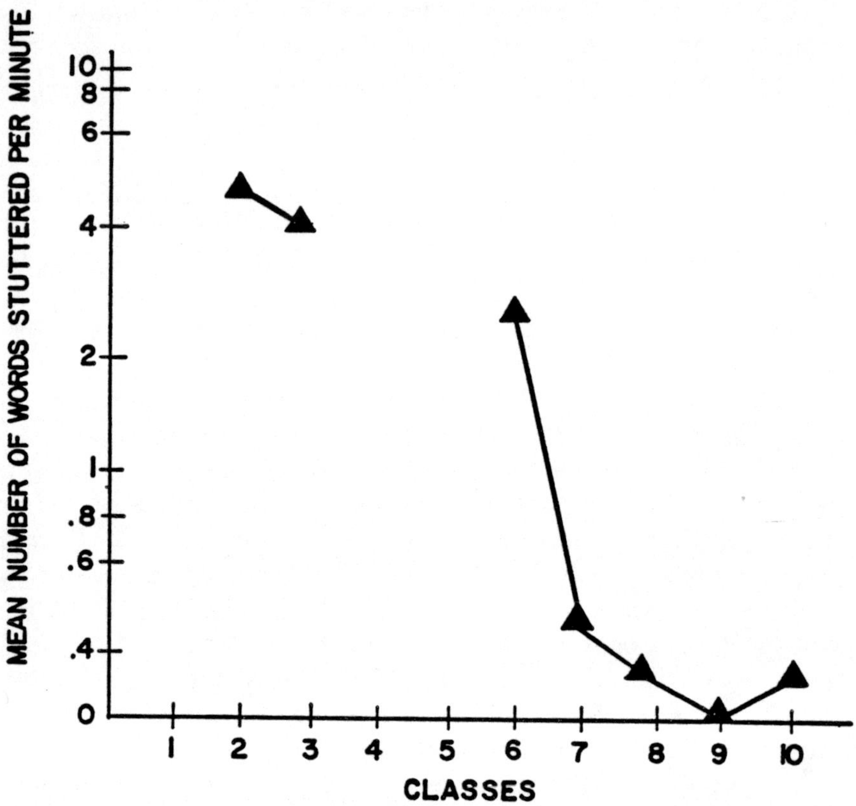

Figure 29. Means of the number of words stuttered per minute for subject HW during the Cough and Smile Classroom Lecture Program.

certain class members were recording his stuttering rate. The next class meeting revealed a rate of 4.0 SW/M.

Subject HW did not lecture during class numbers four and five.

In step two of the program, HW, in the environment of his own office, gave a fifteen-minute monologue to his former therapist, with the instructions, "Do what you do when you want to be fluent." His rate was .07 SW/M. Stuttering rate dropped during the next class period to 2.5 SW/M. During this session, a baseline was also taken on coughing behavior in the classroom. There were .24 coughs per minute. It was felt that this small amount of random coughing would not interfere with using a cough as a consequence in a program.

Coughing behavior was chosen as an aversive stimulus to be used following each stuttered word. The cough was chosen not only for its aversive properties, but also because it was assumed that other class members would not be aware of the use of a cough as a consequence. Smiling contingent upon fluent utterances was also part of the program. HW was informed of the cough-smile consequences, however, the speech pathology students were not pointed out to him.

Teams of two from the fourteen speech pathology students were assigned various fifteen-minute periods during the three-hour class session for "coughing" following a stuttered word. The cough consequence was standardized to a single cough from each person on the team or two simultaneous coughs per team. Concomitant with the cough or punishment, a positive reinforcer of smiling and looking attentive was used during periods of fluency. All fourteen students taking part in the program were engaged in this contingency throughout the class period. Class number seven revealed a great decrease to .4 SW/M.

The next step of the program included fading of the cough consequence to a one-cough event. Criterion was set at .2 SW/M in order to begin this fading. During the second half of the class, criterion was met. The average for the entire class number eight was .34 SW/M.

Additional fading continued in class number nine, with one person coughing after each stuttered word. The positive reinforcers of smiling and attentive behavior were continued throughout the program. Criterion was met and an average of .17 SW/M was recorded for this class.

The report of the project was made to the class at the end of class number nine. The thirty-three nonspeech pathology students in the class were asked to answer a written questionnaire containing the following questions: "What observations have you made about HW's speech throughout the quarter?" and "Have you noticed any extraneous activity in the classroom during the quarter?" Their answers revealed that the class members were aware of the decrease of the stuttering behavior, but were unaware of the existence of the program or its contingencies. Typical answers to question number one were: "Speech much improved; he hasn't stuttered at all for the last three meetings"; and "At the beginning of the term, I noticed a stutter in HW's speech which has in recent weeks stopped." Most of the students answered "no" to question number two regarding extraneous activity during class. Two people had noted what we had hoped was discreet counting of the stuttering rate. And one girl had been annoyed because she had been continually offered cough drops by one of the speech pathology students during the class, in an attempt to keep random coughing rate minimal.

Fading continued during class number ten, with one student coughing after every *other* stuttered word. The cough contingency was completely faded during the second half of the class. A rate of .3 SW/M was recorded for this class.

A change in the topography of the stuttering was noted throughout the program. The stuttering behavior reduced to mild prolongations of short duration and part-word repetitions consisting of a single repetition.

A maintenance program was carried out during the following spring term. HW did not teach any classes that term. Each of eight of the speech pathology students who had taken part in the original modification program was assigned to a particular week in which he or she conversed with HW in at least three different settings. These included a telephone call, conversation in HW's office, and another conversation somewhere in the "real world," such as in a coffee shop, at his home or somewhere on campus. Only some of the students continued the cough-smile contingency throughout the conversations in order to provide for fading. The average stuttering rate for the three conversations was recorded on a large wall graph in HW's office at the end of each week. Stuttering rate during this maintenance program ranged from 0 to .2 SW/M, and averaged less than .1 SW/M.

On one occasion during the spring term, HW lectured to a group of twenty strangers in a different city. Two of the speech pathology students were present, and managed the cough-smile contingency during the lecture. Stuttering rate was .25 SW/M. This indicated that HW was maintaining his low rate even in a different environment than that of the University.

A second maintenance program was carried out during the summer session. Two speech pathology students initiated conversations with HW on an intermittent basis, while continuing the fading of the cough-smile contingency. The rate of SW/M remained below .2 during these conversations. A student who had HW on her dissertation committee reported that he remained fluent during the committee meeting.

Stuttering behavior was thus successfully modified in the classroom situation using a smile-cough contingency for fluency and stuttering, respectively. The resultant stuttering rate of less than .2 SW/M was maintained for at least two terms following the modification program.

Author's Note: "I said they were unusual."

CLIENT'S FAILURE PERFORMANCE

The results of the procedures generally have been positive. Our most recent clients and programs reflect our best efforts and these results look very good (Van Kirk, 1972). There were, however, a number of failures along the way and there is value in sharing them, not only for our own humility, but to help our colleagues avoid some of our errors.

To begin to factor out error, a criterion of success of a rate of less than 1 SW/M was chosen. To further sort through our failures we grouped them into establishment, transfer and maintenance problems.

Establishment Programs

Our earliest efforts were characterized by rather gross programs. We constantly sought the correct criterion levels of time on the program and fluency levels. In our first full year of work we held to a criterion of 1 or less SW/M. This proved possible to accomplish, but the general results as characterized by clients DP, CC, JA and DCo on Program I, Programmed Traditional, were not very encouraging. DCo presented us with an unusual problem of a client who could not verbalize even one sound when in his long blocks. We were unprepared for him and could not find a solution with several months of therapy. He left therapy.

Fortunately, our other results were positive, therefore, in the next year we set the criterion at 0 SW/M and focused on Program 2, Delayed Auditory Feedback, which provided us with a much more powerful Establishment Program. It produced very low rates of stuttering. However, we found that setting the criterion at 0 SW/M for forty minutes was too high. We had several sessions of thirty-nine minutes and fifty-seven seconds at which point one small part-word repetition erased the entire effort. These high criterion levels also forced us to stay in the establishment phase too long. Several clients gave up on us after numerous sessions of reading aloud (DCo, GL). We then went to criterion levels of .5 SW/M for five minutes. These, initially, appeared to be too inefficient as demonstrated by the performance of JS and WH on Program 2, Delayed Auditory Feedback. The SW/M level should have been 0.

We had three additional people drop out of very successful Establishment Programs before they were completed. We were able to find only one of them to interview afterwards and his comments were vague, i.e. he said something about being too busy for therapy. Maybe some people who stutter really want to or at least do not want to pay the price in time and effort to become fluent. Perhaps they are being reinforced for stuttering in their environment.

We also had a few completely valueless Establishment Programs such as trying to reinforce fluent utterances without informing the person while the person was engaging in monologue (Haugen, 1967a). This procedure is not to be confused with Program 4, GILCU. The failure program started too high and the steps were too large.

Another kind of ineffective program was the casual program of occasional visits for therapy, usually intermittent on no set schedule. This was usually in response to people who lived a long distance from the clinic and simply wanted a bit of advice or general treatment suggestions. The author succumbed to this enticement and plea for help from several different people. The evidence was that casual, informal programs did not work. This kind of "counseling" is a waste of both the clinician's time and the client's time.

Another error was in believing that if the clients stored up enough fluency in the clinic (like flying time for a pilot) they would spontaneously transfer their fluency. This may have been true for many of the children, but it did not hold for most of the adults. Long Establishment Programs kept us from more functional transfer procedures.

Our major error was in lack of expertise in program design. We caution our colleagues not to take programmed therapy casually or to try to write or carry out programs without basic programming knowledge. Operant speech therapy is not difficult to carry out once the basic skills have been learned, but those skills of counting stuttered words, timing, reinforcing, writing and following programs, etc. must be well-learned either through extensive self-experience or through training. We eventually did learn, however, to use lower criterion levels and smaller steps which have led to improved programs (Ryan and Van Kirk, 1971).

Transfer Programs

Our major error in Transfer Programs was that we did not start them soon enough or give enough transfer activity. The long term failures of clients WH, SP, TS, and CM are partly due to the lack of adequate Transfer Programs. As we have increased the Transfer Program in scope and criterion levels, the overall effectiveness of maintenance has improved.

It apparently is important to provide *in vivo* experiences in speaking in a number of different situations. We found in recent Transfer Programs that it was necessary to add the special instruction to talk fluently all the time. A special series, the all day, sixteen-hour fluency series, was designed especially to help the clients generalize to all of their everyday speaking.

One failure we made on several occasions in early Transfer Programs was not going into special areas like the client's home or work. Client DC, described in the earlier illustration of Program 3, Punishment, earlier in this chapter, demonstrated another kind of transfer error. We did not make an initial contract with DC to observe him speaking in his school. We should have. Initial contracts or showing the older clients the entire transfer and maintenance sequence and having them agree at least verbally to this sequence has proved helpful. It is probably better not to take clients, if they are unwilling to participate in a Transfer Program. Our present Transfer Program is longer than the Establishment Program and we put everybody through it (Ryan and Van Kirk, 1971).

Maintenance Programs

The same general observations about Transfer Programs may be made about Maintenance Programs. We did not do enough. A major problem is follow-up or maintenance. One of our clients refused a $50.00 bonus for returning some maintenance data. The present major problem in maintenance is getting the clients to continue to participate. As they become fluent they lose interest in taking the time and energy to stay in contact with us. If they fail badly, they are either too embarrassed because they think it is their fault or too angry with us because they think it is our fault, to return. Out of the clients we trained we do not have any follow-up data on twenty-eight of the fifty-eight people (48 per cent) we have had on programs. We must find some way to follow them up or we will never know the true results of our therapy procedures.

There were other types of errors, to be sure, but most of them were human ones like going to the wrong step, etc. The ones just recounted were the common, major errors. We have solved most of these problems. Consistent, long term follow-up remains our single most important problem yet to be solved.

SUMMARY

This chapter gave illustrations of clients going through the four Establishment Programs and some form of Transfer and Maintenance Programs. The clients chosen were successful in achieving speech fluency. They represent the performance of clients going through our present improved program procedures.

The second part of the chapter was composed of client performance in rather unusual programs involving clock clicks, coughing and money contingencies to increase and decrease stuttering behavior.

The final part was devoted to a failure analysis in which it was pointed out that simple ignorance of program design and the lack of extensive Transfer and Maintenance Programs were responsible for most of our early failures.

CHAPTER VIII

SUMMARY

SUMMARY OF CHAPTERS I-VIII

IN CHAPTER I THERE WAS discussion about stuttering as learned behavior. The three major behavioral components of stuttering: anxiety, speech and attitude were described. Basic principles of operant learning theory and their application to stuttering were presented.

Chapter II described and illustrated the basic technology of operant conditioning to describe the stuttering behavior observed and to record the data generated by operant speech fluency programs.

Chapter III showed two test procedures: The Stuttering Interview (SI), one form for children and one form for adults, and the Criterion Test (CT) or Base Rate. These two measures are essential to the running of operant speech fluency programs.

Chapter IV described some of the rules of programming and how they apply to the development of operant speech fluency programs.

Chapter V was composed of description, examples and data on each of the four Establishment Programs: Program 1, Programmed Traditional; Program 2, Delayed Auditory Feedback; Program 3, Punishment; and Program 4, Gradual Increase in Length and Complexity of Utterance. The data shown indicated that each was effective. The four programs were compared.

Chapter VI presented the Transfer and Maintenance Programs which provide for generalization and permanency of fluency evoked in the Establishment Programs. Data were presented and the importance of these two procedures to the total therapy process was emphasized.

Chapter VII presented client performance on the four Establishment Programs, on some unusual programs, and an analysis of clients and programs which failed.

THE GOAL OF FLUENCY PROGRAMS

The emphasis is and should be on fluency. All of the data presented in this book make one point; normal fluency is a reasonable goal for people who stutter. Shames (1970), Rubin and Culatta (1971) and Bar (1971) have recently offered supporting evidence for the achievement of such a target. The programmer always starts the program by describing the end-goal or target behavior. It seems only appropriate that the target be normal, fluent speech. At least the effort should be made. If it is true that there are a wide variety of stutterers and some of them are literally incurable, then this procedure will cause them to be identified very clearly and rather quickly.

Our major problem with the goal of normal fluency is the definition of normal fluency. There is a lack of data about the normal word rate and disfluency rate of normal speakers in normal speaking situations. One program (Van Kirk, 1971) utilized the post-program comparison of the client with two of his or her peers. When the lay judges cannot consistently pick out the ex-stutterer, Van Kirk considers them ready for dismissal. She assumes her client has normal speech. There is great need for normative information on normal fluency rates in reading, monologue and conversation, both in and out of the *clinic* situations.

If we accept the basic premise that normal fluency is a realistic, achievable goal, what does this mean to the clinician who stutters? Functionally, it does not change the situation very much. The clinician who stutters can carry out most of the operant speech fluency programs described in this book with little or no difficulty except perhaps in those procedures which require fluent modeling or, fluent conversational partners. It does seem reasonable, however, that a clinician running a successful operant speech fluency program which is helping many clients achieve normal fluency would also want to achieve such fluency. The important point is that the clinician who stutters has the opportunity now, through operant speech fluency programs, to become fluent. The clinician may also choose to continue to stutter.

UNIVERSAL PROGRAMS

This book has demonstrated a wide variety of programs (four Establishment Programs, several Transfer and Maintenance Programs, and some programs which defy title). Program 2, Delayed Auditory Feedback, has been run in much the same way on a very large number of people. Its effects are universal. Is there one universal program for the treatment of stuttering such as the omnibus program described in Chapter V? If there is, will everybody use it? There are at least four universal Establishment Programs which have been demonstrated to be very effective. Only further research will answer the question as to whether or not one is better than the others, or if an omnibus program is better than any of the four. The Transfer and Maintenance Programs do seem universal. As to whether or not everyone would use them, that is a much more difficult question to answer. In today's mobile society it certainly would be very helpful if similar programs were being run across the country. Not only could the client who moves continue on the same helpful program (at the same step, even) in a new location, but there would also be a system for follow-up which would provide us with valuable maintenance information so badly needed at this time.

One final advantage of universal programs would be that the probability of building a program which would be especially efficient and helpful would be increased because so many people would be cooperatively gathering data on it and helping to refine it.

CRITICISMS OF OPERANT SPEECH FLUENCY THERAPY

There has been some criticism of operant speech fluency programs. Most of the criticism comes from either uninformed people or people with vested interest in other theoretical positions concerning stuttering. Most of the criticisms fall into at least one of the following four categories.

Operant Speech Fluency Therapy Is Ineffective

Critics say that it is ineffective because it does not deal with the real problem (anxiety, self-concept, role-conflict, anal regression, oral aggression, morale). Most of the people I have worked with who stutter described the real problem as, "I stutter." This statement commonly refers to their speech. The clients who refer to other problems are usually people who have had extensive speech therapy elsewhere, previously. Even if the achievement of speech fluency alone does not solve all of the person's problems, it at least solves one of them.

Others say it is not effective because it produces only laboratory fluency. This criticism may have been true of the early work in operant speech fluency programs. The early work was mostly of a laboratory demonstration nature. However, the programs have become more sophisticated in the past few years and at present do deal with both transfer to the outside world and with the maintenance of the fluency.

We do need more information about the interaction among speech fluency, anxiety and attitude. Although much of our experience has been that speech fluency produces improved attitudes, which is supported by the work of Martin and Haroldson (1969) and Shames (1970), much more data are needed. The data we presently have on the relationship between speech fluency and anxiety are inconsistent (Gray and England, 1972). Perhaps the answer lies in a combined approach of fluency training and attitude change such as that reported by Blind, Shames and Egolf (1971).

The real measure of effectiveness awaits mutual agreement on the target of stuttering therapy. At present, the data indicate that operant speech fluency programs produce speech fluency very effectively and that at least one target should be normal, human fluent speech.

Operant Speech Fluency Therapy Is the Rediscovery of Some Old Bogus Procedures

This criticism is leveled in two ways. The first is that operant therapy programs have merely rediscovered Benjamin Bogus and put him in new clothes especially with all the emphasis on the practice of fluent speech. While it is probably true that if Mr. Bogus had known anything about operant technology he probably would have doubled his fortune, the present procedures are really quite different from anything that would have been found going on in his office. This criticism appears to be more a semantic game of a condemnation by linking the two procedures together rather than any criticism based on fact.

The second is that operant procedures are merely distraction procedures which produce temporary fluency (Biggs and Sheehan, 1969). This also is an example of condemnation by labelling. Distraction, as described in the literature, appears to be any procedure such as finger snapping or talking in an accent or sighing which produces *temporary* fluency. The implication is that distraction is ineffective. Therefore, labelling operant procedures as distraction procedures now makes them, by semantic fiat, ineffective. From the operant point of view any number of procedures including those mentioned above can be stimulus supports to evoke fluency. The gradual withdrawal of these supports is critical to the maintenance of the behavior. Previous studies viewed numerous procedures as distractions in either-or situations and consequently condemned them for failure to produce permanent fluency. There was no effort to gradually fade them. In addition, if we define distraction as a set of procedures which produces only temporary fluency then we say that most common therapy procedures have been nothing more than distractions (Prins, 1969; Gregory, 1969; Van Riper, 1958) because none of them has produced permanent lasting changes in speech fluency in any large number of clients.

Operant Speech Fluency Therapy Is Pseudo-Scientific

The major critical point is that all the counting and charting and use of the word, *data,* do not make a scientific approach. That criticism is partly right. It is the correct use of counting, charting and *data* that is scientific. The problem is to decide where science begins and pseudo-science ends. If what we are doing is not science, then at least it is a closer approximation than not collecting any data at all. In addition, this criticism should be applied not only to operant procedures but to any therapy process. We, all, must attempt to become as accurate and precise as we can in dealing with the very difficult problem of stuttering. Our experience with the data collection procedures described in this book has taught us both a respect for the rigors of science (it is very difficult to meet all the standards) and an appreciation for the measurement and precision of therapy management which is built into operant therapy programs. We have lost interest in discussing those procedures which do not have data to support their efficiency.

Operant Speech Fluency Therapy Is Cold and Mechanical

The critics, usually humanists, state that no human being is really helped by having his dignity destroyed by learning how to speak fluently. Apparently, these critics are responding to the operant literature which described people as subjects and which very carefully attempted to control both the human interaction variables and the manipulation of the subjects. These efforts at a science of human behavior apparently have been interpreted as the only way operant therapy programs can or are ever carried out.

All of the programs described in this book were carried out in settings which contained two human beings talking and/or listening to each other. The critical difference between the two people was that one was following a prescribed programmed procedure. The major observation made by most people who observed our operant therapy programs is that the client seems to be doing all the reading or talking. The second most common observation is that the client is very fluent. "Does he really stutter?" is a question asked by those who observe after the first day of therapy. Our clinical therapy programs described in this book are really quite humanistic. We like the people we work with and we express it to them. What is even more humanistic is the response from the client. Our clients and their parents or spouses have generally been warm, sensitive people who genuinely appreciate becoming fluent through their interaction with us. I could fill the rest of this book with testimonials (two are on video-tape). The problem apparently is that the critics are responding to a few examples in the literature with almost no personal observation of the procedures. The critics may also be responding to examples of some operant procedures which are quite different from those described in this book.

Actually, this entire book is presented as an answer to the criticism raised against operant speech fluency practices. All of us interested in helping people who stutter must first communicate with each other. Secondly, we must agree on the ground rules and target behaviors for people who stutter. I suggest that speech fluency be at least one. Finally, we must be willing to share data, in some form, as I have tried to do in this book. The data will bring the truth. The truth will help us develop effective strategies for the treatment of stuttering.

RESEARCH

The discussion of research needs must be circumscribed to those areas discussed in this book. There is great need of research. The first is to refine all the procedures and programs which have been described in this book. Each of the programs must be continually evaluated and revised to provide the most effective treatment system possible. Fortunately, the data collection is built into the operant system and we are presently gathering data on all of these programs with the goal of improvement.

A second research effort should go into comparing the four different Establishment Programs. We should find the best one or ones.

A third major area is the study of normal human fluency and the accumulation of important normative data on speech rates of normal speakers in reading, monologue and conversation. We must define our target behavior.

A fourth area is the study of the development of stuttering in preschool children. Our work has extended down to three-year-olds, but we did not do much other than observe them in diagnostic evaluations with the SI and recommend simple home procedures. A major area of interest and need is the behavioral study of stimuli, responses and consequences of the interaction between the child and his parents and siblings. We have the tools via the operant system. Such research is exemplified by the interesting work of Wahler, Sperling, Thomas, Teeter and Luper (1970) to study and change home situations to eliminate the problem of stuttering.

A WORD OF CAUTION

No one should try to carry out the programs described in this book without careful consideration of the skills brought to the task. Such "do it yourself" operant speech fluency training may be responsible for much criticism of the approach. One should not attempt to put these programs into action without first careful study and preparation. The skills described in Chapter II must be mastered first. Special training may be necessary. One should practice on normal speakers first. It is especially important that thc programs not be dissected or used in pieces. They are designed to run as written, in the sequence and with the reinforcing events outlined, as a carefully structured clinical tool.

A POSITIVE FINAL NOTE

The data in this book and those that are being collected across the country in clinics, clinic-laboratories and laboratories are very encouraging. It may well be that we finally discovered a problem solving system which will help us solve the problem of stuttering.

BIBLIOGRAPHY

Adamczyk, B.: Use of instruments for the production of artificial feedback in the treatment of stuttering. *Folia Phoniatr, 11*:216-218, 1959.

Andrews, G., and Harris, M.: The Syndrome of Stuttering. Clinics in developmental medicine, No. 17. London, Heinemann, 1964.

Andrews, G., and Ingham, R.: Stuttering: The quality of fluency after treatment. Paper presented at the Annual Convention, American Speech and Hearing Association, Chicago, November, 1971.

Ayllon, T., and Azrin, N.: *The Token Economy: A Motivational System for Therapy and Rehabilitation*. New York, Appleton, 1968.

Azrin, N., Jones, R., and Flye, B.: A synchronization effect and its application to stuttering by a portable apparatus. *J Applied Behavior Analysis, 1*: 283-295, 1968.

Bandura, A.: *Principles of Behavior Modification*. New York, HR&W, 1969.

Bar, A.: The shaping of fluency, not the modification of stuttering. *J Commun Disord, 4*:1-7, 1971.

Beech, H., and Fransella, F.: *Research and Experiment in Stuttering*. Oxford, Pergamon, 1968.

Biggs, B., and Sheehan, J.: Punishment or distraction? Operant-stuttering revisited. *J Abnorm Psychol, 74*:256-262, 1969.

Blind, J., Shames, G., and Egolf, D.: The combined use of operant procedures and theoretical concepts in the treatment of an adult female stutterer. *J Speech Hear Disord, 36*:414-421, 1971.

Bradfield, R. (Ed.): *Behavior Modification of Learning Disabilities*. San Rafael, Academic Therapy Publications, 1971.

Brady, J.: Studies on the metronome effect on stuttering. *Behav Res Ther, 7*: 197-204, 1969.

Branch, R., and Sulzbacher, S.: Rapid computation of rates with a simple nomogram. *J Applied Behavior Analysis, 1*:251, 1968.

Brookshire, R.: Speech pathology and the experimental analysis of behavior. *J Speech Hear Disord, 32*:215-227, 1967.

Brutten, G., and Shoemaker, D.: Behavior check list. Carbondale, Southern Illinois University, 1970.

Brutten, G., and Shoemaker, D.: *The Modification of Stuttering*. Englewood Cliffs, P-H, 1967.

Chase, R., Sutton, S., and Rapin, I.: Sensory feedback influences on motor performance. *J Auditory Research, 3*:212-223, 1961.

Cherry, C., and Sayers, B.: Experiments upon total inhibition of stammering by external control and some clinical results. *J Psychosom Res, 1*:233-246, 1956.

Cooper, E., Cady, B., and Robbins, C.: The effect of the verbal stimulus words "wrong, right" and "tree" on the dysfluency rates of stutterers and non-stutterers. *J Speech Hear Res, 13*:229-244, 1970.

Cram, D.: *Explaining Teaching Machines and Programming.* San Francisco, Fearon, 1961.

Curlee, R., and Perkins, W.: Conversational rate control therapy for stuttering. *J Speech Hear Disord, 34*:245-250, 1969.

Daly, D., and Frick, J.: The effects of punishing stuttering expectations and stuttering utterances: A comparative study. *Behav Ther, 1*:228-239, 1970.

Edling, J.: *Individualized Instruction: A Manual for Administrators.* Corvallis, Division of Continuing Education, 1969.

Egolf, D., Shames, G., and Seltzer, H.: The effects of time-out on the fluency of stutterers in group therapy. *J Commun Disord, 4*:111-118, 1971.

Egolf, D., Shames, G., Johnson, P., and Kasprisin-Burrelli, A.: The use of parent-child interactions patterns in therapy for young stutterers. *J Speech Hear Disord, 37*:222-232, 1972.

Eisenson, J.: A perseverative theory of stuttering. In Eisenson, J. (Ed.): *Stuttering: A Symposium.* New York, Har-Row, 1958.

Espich, J., and Williams, B.: *Developing Programmed Instructional Materials.* Palo Alto, Fearon, 1967.

Fairbanks, G.: *Voice and Articulation.* New York, Har-Row, 1960.

Fargo, G., and Behrns, C.: Rapid computation and pupil self-recording of performance data. *J Applied Behavior Analysis, 2*:264, 1969.

Fargo, G., Behrns, C., and Nolen, P.: *Behavior Modification in the Classroom.* Belmont, Wadsworth Pub, 1970.

Felty, J.: *The operant nature of stuttering behavior of adolescent boys,* Unpublished master's thesis, Seattle, University of Washington, 1959.

Flanagan, B., Goldiamond, I., and Azrin, N.: Operant stuttering: The control of stuttering behavior through response-contingent consequences. *J Exp Anal Behav, 1*:173-177, 1958.

Fransella, F., and Beech, H.: An experimental analysis of the effect of rhythm on the speech of stutterers. *Behav Res Ther, 3*:195-201, 1965.

Fraser, M. (Ed.): *Conditioning in Stuttering Therapy: Applications and Limitations.* Memphis, Speech Foundation of America, 1970.

Fraser, M. (Ed.): *Treatment of the Young Stutterer in the School.* Memphis, Speech Foundation of America, 1964.

Girardeau, F., and Spradlin, J.: A functional analysis approach to speech and language. *American Speech and Hearing Association Monographs,* No. 14, 1970.

Goldiamond, I.: Blocked speech communication and delayed feedback: An experimental design. Technical report no. 1, progress report, Operational

Applications Laboratory, Air Force Cambridge Research Center, Bedford, 1960a.

Goldiamond, I.: Effects of delayed feedback upon the temporal development of fluent and blocked speech communication. Technical report, No. 2. Operational Applications Laboratory, Air Force Cambridge Research Center, Bedford, 1960b.

Goldiamond, I.: Stuttering and fluency as manipulatable operant response classes. In Krasner, L., and Ullman, L. (Eds.): *Research in Behavior Modification*. New York, HR&W, 1965.

Goldiamond, I.: The maintenance of ongoing fluent verbal behavior and stuttering. *J Mathetics, 1*:57-95, 1962.

Goldiamond, I.: The temporal development of fluent and blocked speech communication. Final report and technical reports, Nos. 2, 3, 4. Operational Applications Laboratory, Air Force Cambridge Research Center, Bedford, 1960c.

Gray, B.: Some effects of anxiety deconditioning upon stuttering. Final report, research and demonstration project 2021-S, Social and Rehabilitation Service, U.S. Department of Health, Education and Welfare, Washington, D.C., 1969.

Gray, B., and England, G.: Some effects of anxiety deconditioning upon stuttering frequency. *J Speech Hear Res, 15*:114-121, 1972.

Gray, B., and England, G. (Eds.): *Stuttering and the Conditioning Therapies*. Monterey, Monterey Institute of Speech and Hearing, 1969.

Gray, B., and Fygetakis, L.: Mediated language acquisition for dysphasic children. *Behav Res Ther, 6*:263-280, 1968.

Greenberg, J.: The effect of a metronome on the speech of young stutterers. *Behav Ther, 1*:240-244, 1970.

Gregory, H.: An assessment of the results of stuttering therapy. Final report, research and demonstration project 1725-S, Social and Rehabilitation Service, U.S. Department of Health, Education and Welfare, Washington, D.C., 1969.

Gregory, H.: *Learning Theory and Stuttering Therapy*. Evanston, Northwestern U Pr, 1968.

Griffin, K., and Van Kirk, B.: Modification of stuttering behavior in a natural environment. Paper presented at the Annual Convention, American Speech and Hearing Association, Chicago, November, 1969.

Gross, M., and Holland, A.: The effects of response contingent electroshock upon stuttering. *ASHA, 7*:376-377, 1965.

Gross, M., and Gregory, H.: The use of operant conditioning procedures in conjunction with a more traditional stuttering therapy program. Paper presented at the Annual Convention, American Speech and Hearing Association, Washington, D.C., November, 1966.

Gross, M., and Nathanson, S.: A study of the use of a DAF procedure for adult stutterers. Paper presented at the Annual Convention, American Speech and Hearing Association, Chicago, November, 1967.

Gruber, L.: The use of the portable voice masker in stuttering therapy. *J Speech Hear Disord, 36*:287-289, 1971.

Hahn, E., Lomas, C., Hargis, D., and Vandraegen, D.: *Basic Voice Training for Speech*. New York, McGraw, 1952.

Halvorson, J.: The effects on stuttering frequency of pairing punishment (response cost) with reinforcement. *J Speech Hear Res, 14*:356-364, 1971.

Ham, R., and Steer, M.: Certain effects of alterations in auditory feedback. *Folia Phoniatr, 19*:53-62, 1967.

Haroldson, S., Martin, R., and Starr, C.: Time-out as a punishment of stuttering. *J Speech Hear Res, 11*:560-566, 1968.

Haugen, D.: *An experimental clinical procedure for modifying stuttering behavior in a child*. Unpublished paper, Eugene, University of Oregon, 1967a.

Haugen, D.: *The clinical application of a program for modifying stuttering behavior*. Unpublished paper, Eugene, University of Oregon, 1967b.

Holland, A.: Some applications of behaviorial principles to clinical speech problems. *J Speech Hear Disord, 32*:11-18, 1967.

Holland, J., and Skinner, B.: *The Analysis of Behavior*. New York, McGraw, 1961.

Honig, W. (Ed.): *Operant Behavior: Areas of Research and Application*. New York, Appleton, 1966.

Hood, S.: *Clinical assessment of the moment of stuttering*. Unpublished paper, Bowling Green, Bowling Green State University, 1971.

Ingham, R., and Andrews, J.: Stuttering: A description and analysis of a token economy in an adult therapy programme. Paper presented at the Annual Convention, American Speech and Hearing Association, Chicago, November, 1971.

Johnson, W.: Measures of oral reading and speaking rate and disfluency of adult male and female stutterers and nonstutterers. Studies of speech disfluency and rate of stutterers and nonstutterers. *J Speech Hear Disord*, Monograph Supplement No. *7*:1-20, 1961.

Johnson, W. (Ed.): *Stuttering in Children and Adults*. Minneapolis, U of Minn Pr, 1955.

Johnson, W., Brown, M., Curtis, J., and Keaster, J.: *Speech Handicapped School Children*. New York, Har-Row, 1956.

Johnston, J.: A universal behavior graph paper. *J Applied Behavior Analysis, 3*:271, 1970.

Jones, R., and Azrin, N.: Behavioral engineering: Stuttering as a function of stimulus duration during speech synchronization. *J Applied Behavior Analysis, 2*:223-230, 1969.

Krasner, L., and Ullmann, L. (Eds.): *Research in Behavior Modification, New Developments and Implications.* New York, HR&W, 1965.

Lanyon, R.: Behavior change in stuttering through systematic desensitization. *J Speech Hear Disord, 34:*253-260, 1969.

Leach, E.: Stuttering: Clinical application of response-contingent procedures. In Gray, B., and England, G. (Eds.): *Stuttering and the Conditioning Therapies.* Monterey, Monterey Institute for Speech and Hearing, 1969.

Lindsley, O.: Daily behavior chart (DC-8) 6 cycle-140 days (20 wks.), Kansas City, Behavior Research Co., 1968.

Logue, R.: *The effects of temporal alteration in auditory feedback upon the speech output of stutterers and non-stutterers.* Unpublished master's thesis, West Lafayette, Purdue University, 1962.

Lotzmann, G.: Zue annendung varuerter versogerungszeiten bei balbuties. *Folia Phoniatr, 13:*276-312, 1961.

Luper, H., and Mulder, R.: *Stuttering: Therapy for Children.* Englewood Cliffs, P-H, 1964.

Mager, R.: *Preparing Instructional Objectives.* Palo Alto, Fearon, 1962.

Markle, S.: *Good Frames and Bad, a Grammar of Frame Writing.* New York, Wiley, 1964.

Martin, R.: The experimental manipulation of stuttering behaviors. In Sloane, H., and MacAulay, B. (Eds.): *Operant Procedures in Remedial Speech and Language Training.* New York, HM, 1968.

Martin, R., and Berndt, L.: The effects of time-out on stuttering in a 12-year-old boy. *Except Child, 37:*303-304, 1970.

Martin, R., and Haroldson, S.: The effects of two treatment procedures on stuttering. *J Commun Disord, 2:*115-125, 1969.

Martin, R., and Haroldson, S.: Time-out as a punishment for stuttering during conversation. *J Commun Disord, 4:*15-19, 1971.

Martin, R., Haroldson, S., and Starr, C.: Time-out as punishment for stuttering: A reply to Martin Adams. Letters to the editor, *J Speech Hear Res, 14:*220-222, 1971.

Martin, R., and Siegel, G.: The effects of response contingent shock on stuttering. *J Speech Hear Res, 9:*340-352, 1966a.

Martin, R., and Siegel, G.: The effects of simultaneously punishing stuttering and rewarding fluency. *J Speech Hear Res, 9:*466-475, 1966b.

Meyer, V., and Comley, J.: A preliminary report on the treatment of stammer by the use of rhythmic stimulation. In Gray, B., and England, G. (Eds.): *Stuttering and the Conditioning Therapies.* Monterey, Monterey Institute for Speech and Hearing, 1969.

Meyer, V., and Mair, J.: A new technique to control stammering: a preliminary report. *Behav Res Ther, 1:*251-254, 1963.

Mowrer, D.: Evaluating speech therapy through precision recording. *J Speech Hear Disord, 34:*239-244, 1969.

Mowrer, D.: Speech response chart. Salt Lake City, Word Making Productions, Inc., 1971a.

Mowrer, D.: Technical research report S-1: Reduction of stuttering behavior. Tempe, The Arizona State University Bookstore, 1971b.

Mowrer, D.: Transfer of training in articulation therapy. *J Speech Hear Disord, 36:*427-446, 1971c.

Murray, F.: An investigation of variably induced white noise upon moments of stuttering. *J Commun Disord, 2:*109-114, 1969.

Naylor, R.: A comparative study of methods of estimating the severity of stuttering. *J Speech Hear Disord, 18:*30-37, 1953.

Neelley, J.: A study of the speech behavior of stutterers and nonstutterers under normal and delayed auditory feedback. *J Speech Hear Disord.* Monograph Supplement No. 7:63-82, 1961.

Peins, M., Lee, B., and McGough, E.: A tape-recorded method for stutterers: a case study. *J Speech Hear Disord, 35:*188-193, 1970.

Perkins, W.: Modification of stuttering by rate control. Final report, research and demonstration project 2180-S, Vocational Rehabilitation Administration, U.S. Department of Health, Education and Welfare, Washington, D.C., 1967.

Perkins, W., and Curlee, R.: Clinical impressions of portable masking unit effects in stuttering. *J Speech Hear Disord, 34:*360-362, 1969.

Pipe, P.: *Practical Programming.* New York, HR&W, 1966.

Prins, D.: Improvement and regression in stutterers following short-term intensive therapy. *J Speech Hear Disord, 35:*123-134, 1970.

Quist, R., and Martin, R.: The effect of response contingent verbal punishment on stuttering. *J Speech Hear Res, 10:*795-800, 1967.

Rhodes, R., Shames, G., and Egolf, D.: "Awareness" in verbal conditioning of language themes during therapy with stutterers. *J Speech Hear Disord, 4:*30-39, 1971.

Rickard, H., and Mundy, M.: Direct manipulation of stuttering behavior, an experimental-clinical approach. In Ullmann, L., and Krasner, L. (Eds.): *Case Studies in Behavior Modification.* New York, HR&W, 1965.

Rubin, H., and Culatta, R.: A point of view about fluency. *ASHA, 13:*380-389, 1971.

Ryan, B.: An illustration of operant conditioning therapy for stuttering. In Fraser, M. (Ed.): *Conditioning in Stuttering Therapy: Applications and Limitations.* Memphis, Speech Foundation of America, 1970a.

Ryan, B.: *Behavior modification applied to the problem of stuttering children and adults.* Unpublished paper, Monterey, Monterey Institute for Speech and Hearing, 1970b.

Ryan, B.: The effects of positive reinforcement on the frequency of stuttering behavior. Paper presented at the Annual Convention, American Speech and Hearing Association, Chicago, November, 1967.

Ryan, B.: Operant procedures applied to stuttering therapy for children. *J Speech Hear Disord, 36:*264-280, 1971.

Ryan, B.: *The construction and evaluation of a program for modifying stuttering behavior.* Unpublished doctoral dissertation, Pittsburgh, University of Pittsburgh, 1964.

Ryan, B.: The establishment, transfer and maintenance of fluent reading and speaking in a stutterer using operant technology. Paper presented at the Annual Convention, American Speech and Hearing Association, Denver, November, 1968a.

Ryan, B.: The use of DAF in the establishment of fluent reading and speaking in six stutterers. Paper presented at the Annual Convention, American Speech and Hearing Association, Denver, November, 1968b.

Ryan, B., and Shames, G.: The construction and evaluation of a program for modifying stuttering behavior employing operant conditioning principles. Paper presented at the Annual Convention, American Speech and Hearing Association, Washington, D.C., November, 1966.

Ryan, B., and Van Kirk, B.: Counting disfluencies, stuttered words, and total words. A tape recorded training program, Monterey, Monterey Learning Systems, 1973.

Ryan, B., and Van Kirk, B.: Programmed Conditioning for Fluency: Program Book. Monterey, Monterey Learning Systems, 1971.

Shames, G.: Operant conditioning and stuttering. In Gray, B., and England, G. (Eds.): *Stuttering and the Conditioning Therapies.* Monterey, Monterey Institute for Speech and Hearing, 1969a.

Shames, G.: Operant conditioning and therapy for stuttering. In Fraser, M. (Ed.): *Conditioning in Stuttering Therapy: Applications and Limitations.* Memphis, Speech Foundation of America, 1970.

Shames, G.: Verbal reinforcement during therapy interviews. In Gray, B., and England, G. (Eds.): *Stuttering and the Conditioning Therapies.* Monterey, Monterey Institute for Speech and Hearing, 1969b.

Shames, G.: Personal communication, 1971.

Shames, G., and Egolf, D.: Experimental therapy for school-age children and their parents. Progress report, Office of Education project 0-8-0800080-3525, U.S. Department of Health, Education and Welfare, Washington, D.C., 1970.

Shames, G., Egolf, D., and Rhodes, R.: Experimental programs in stuttering therapy. *J Speech Hear Disord, 34:*30-47, 1969.

Shames, G., Lingwall, J., Bryden, J., Rowe, C., Case, J., Blythe, T., Calhoun, R., Sheehy, B., Costello, J., and Ryan, B.: Taos Index of Disfluency (TID). *Feedback, 1:*11-12, 1970.

Shames, G., and Sherrick, C., Jr.: A discussion of nonfluency and stuttering as operant behavior. *J Speech Hear Disord, 28:*3-17, 1963.

Shames, G., and Sherrick, C., Jr.: A discussion of nonfluency and stuttering as operant behavior. In Barbara, D. (Ed.): *New Directions in Stuttering.* Springfield, Thomas, 1965.

Shaw, C., and Shrum, W.: The effects of response-contingent reward on the connected speech of children who stutter. *J Speech Hear Disord, 37*:75-88, 1972.

Sheehan, J.: Conflict theory of stuttering. In Eisenson, J. (Ed.): *Stuttering: A Symposium.* New York, Har-Row, 1959.

Sheehan, J. (Ed.): *Stuttering: Research and Therapy.* New York, Har-Row, 1970.

Sheehan, J.: The modification of stuttering through nonreinforcement. *J Abnorm Psychol, 46*:51-63, 1951.

Sheehan, J., and Voas, R.: Stuttering as conflict: A comparison of therapy techniques involving approach and avoidance. *J Speech Hear Disord, 22*: 714-723, 1957.

Sidman, M.: Operant techniques. In Bachrach, A. (Ed.): *Experimental Foundations of Clinical Psychology.* New York, Basic, 1962.

Siegel, G.: Punishment, stuttering and disfluency. *J Speech Hear Disord, 13*: 677-714, 1970.

Silverman, E.: Evaluating preschoolers' disfluency. *Ohio J Speech Hear, 6*:87-91, 1971a.

Silverman, E.: Situational variability of preschoolers' disfluency: Preliminary study. *Percept Mot Skills, 33*:1021-1022, 1971b.

Silverman, E.: The influence of preschoolers' language usage on their fluency frequency. Paper presented at the Annual Convention, American Speech and Hearing Association, Chicago, November, 1971c.

Silverman, R.: *How to Write a Program: A Programmed Course Designed to Teach Techniques for Programming Instruction.* Carlisle, Carlisle, 1970.

Skinner, B.: *The Behavior of Organisms: An Experimental Analysis.* New York, Appleton, 1938.

Skinner, B.: *Science and Human Behavior.* New York, Macmillan, 1953.

Skinner, B.: *Verbal Behavior.* New York, Appleton, 1957.

Sloane, H., and MacAulay, B. (Eds.) : *Operant Procedures in Remedial Speech and Language Training.* New York, HM, 1969.

Soderberg, G.: Delayed auditory feedback and stuttering. *J Speech Hear Disord, 33*:260-267, 1968.

Soderberg, G.: Delayed auditory feedback and the speech of stutterers: A review of studies. *J Speech Hear Disord, 34*:20-29, 1969.

Soderberg, G.: *A study of the effects of delayed auditory side-tone on four aspects of stutterer's speech during oral reading and spontaneous speaking.* Unpublished doctoral dissertation, Columbus, Ohio State University, 1959.

Thompson, J., and Carlston, H.: The percentage finder. Salt Lake City, 1961.

Toomey, G., and Sidman, M.: An experimental analogue of the anxiety-stuttering relationship. *J Speech Hear Res, 13*:122-129, 1970.

Trotter, W., and Lesch, M.: Personal experiences with a stutter-aid. *J Speech Hear Disord, 32*:270-272, 1967.

Ullmann, L., and Krasner, L. (Eds.): *Case Studies in Behavior Modification.* New York, HR&W, 1965.

Van Kirk, B.: A look at fluency programs with adults over 50 years of age. *Feedback, 2*:6-7, 1970.

Van Kirk, B.: Personal communication, 1971.

Van Kirk, B.: Operant therapy programs for stuttering conducted in a rehabilitation center. *Rehabil Lit, 33*:107-108, 1972.

Van Riper, C.: Experiments in stuttering therapy. In Eisenson, J. (Ed.): *Stuttering: A Symposium.* New York, Har-Row, 1958.

Van Riper, C.: *The Nature of Stuttering.* Englewood Cliffs, P-H, 1971.

Van Riper, C.: *Speech Correction, Principles and Methods.* New York, P-H, 1939.

Van Riper, C.: *Speech Correction, Principles and Methods,* 2nd ed. Englewood Cliffs, P-H, 1947.

Van Riper, C.: *Speech Correction, Principles and Methods,* 3rd ed. Englewood Cliffs, P-H, 1954.

Van Riper, C.: *Speech Correction, Principles and Methods,* 4th ed. Englewood Cliffs, P-H, 1963.

Wahler, R., Sperling, K., Thomas, M., Teeter, N., and Luper, H.: The modification of childhood stuttering: Some response relationships. *J Exp Child Psychol, 3*:411-428, 1970.

Webster, R., and Dorman, M.: Decrease in stuttering frequency as a function of continuous and contingent forms of auditory masking. *J Speech Hear Res, 13*:82-86, 1970.

Webster, R., Schumacher, S., and Lubker, B.: Changes in stuttering frequency as a function of various intervals of delayed auditory feedback. *J Abnorm Psychol, 75*:45-49, 1970.

Wepman, J., and McFarland, R.: Treatment of stammering through the use of a new electronic device. Final report, cooperative research project S-315, U.S. Department of Health, Education and Welfare, Washington, D.C., 1967.

Williams, D.: Modifications of stuttering behavior by use of electric shock. Abstract of convention paper, *ASHA, 4*:408, 1962.

Williams, D.: Stuttering therapy for children. Unpublished paper, Iowa City, University of Iowa, 1970.

Wingate, M.: A standard definition of stuttering. *J Speech Hear Disord, 29*: 484-489, 1964.

Wingate, M.: Calling attention to stuttering. *J Speech Hear Res, 2*:326-335, 1959.

Wingate, M.: Sound and pattern in "artificial" fluency. *J Speech Hear Res, 12*:677-686, 1969.

Wolpe, J.: *Psychotherapy by Reciprocal Inhibition*. Stanford, Stanford U Pr, 1958.

Wolpe, J.: *The Practice of Behavior Therapy*. New York, Pergamon, 1969.

Yates, A.: *Behavior Therapy*. New York, Wiley, 1970.

Yates, A.: Recent empirical and theoretical approaches to the experimental manipulation of speech in normal subjects and in stammerers. *Behav Res Ther, 1*:95-119, 1963.

Yates, A.: The relationship between theory and therapy in the clinical treatment of stuttering. In Gray, B., and England, G. (Eds.): *Stuttering and the Conditioning Therapies*. Monterey, Monterey Institute for Speech and Hearing, 1969.

AUTHOR INDEX

SUBJECT INDEX

U

W